DISEASES OF THE DIGESTIVE SYSTEM

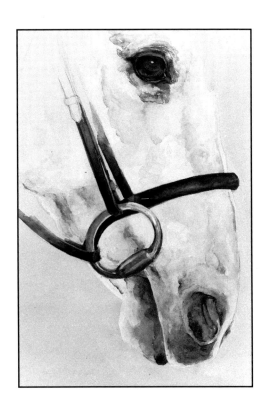

DISEASES OF THE DIGESTIVE SYSTEM

Peter Gray
MVB, MRCVS

J. A. Allen
London

British Library Cataloguing in Publication Data
A catalogue record for this book is available from the British Library

ISBN 0–85131–7170

Published in Great Britain in 1998 by
J. A. Allen & Company Limited
1 Lower Grosvenor Place
London SW1W 0EL

Production editor: Bill Ireson
Illustrator: Maggie Raynor
Cover designer: Nancy Lawrence
Printed in Hong Kong

*To David
whose belated arrival
might, hopefully, herald a new era.
With any luck!*

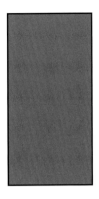

Contents

5 Ingredients of Food   61

6 Defences Against Disease   81

7 Signs of Disease   87

8 Diagnosis and Treatment   92

9 Non-infectious Diseases   111

12 Digestive Diseases of the Foal   165

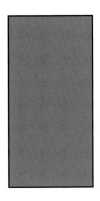

Acknowledgements

My thanks to the following: Brendan Paterson, BVetMed, CertESM, MRCVS, for his help with the manuscript and for providing photographic opportunities; David Byron of MSD AGVET, for again allowing me the use of the parasitology photographs in Chapters 6 and 11; Ian Mole of Equine Marketing, for the use of his two photographs on page 57; Andrew Carter for his photography; Maggie Raynor for the illustrations artwork; my publishers for their continued forbearance. And, finally, thanks to Bill Ireson for his production editing.

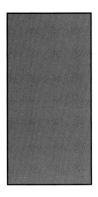

Introduction

The equine digestive system is similar to that of other single-stomached animals – such as the dog – and is designed by nature to ingest, digest and excrete the waste of a diet based on available food from a source outside human control.

The horse is herbivorous, meaning that its appropriate food material is based on grass, plants and plant products. Under the various systems of domestication which the horse today experiences, this food base is expanded to include cereals and, especially in the last few years, a whole range of new products. These products are possibly asking questions of the equine digestive system for which it was never intended. Whether or not this approach leads to disease often depends on management and on a detailed understanding of the working requirements of the system nature created.

The equine digestive system begins with the organs of prehension (that is, the process of taking food into the mouth) and is continued through a succession of (what can be described as) tubular organs. Food material is digested and absorbed in these organs and, eventually, the waste is expelled from the rectum. The system is, thus, a complex structure, consisting of: the mouth (housing the tongue and teeth); the pharynx (throat); oesophagus (gullet); stomach; and small and large intestines – the latter two being further divided by anatomy, position and function within the overall process.

Several structures are associated with the foregoing; for example, the salivary glands and pancreas, which produce secretions vital to digestion. The liver is intimately involved and plays a critical part in the post-absorption processes involving protein, carbohydrate and fat digestion. While these substances are brought to it directly from the bowel, the liver itself is involved in their use within the body – also producing bile which helps the absorption of fat and has other influences on the digestive processes. The liver, too, is one of the principle organs of detoxification, and plays a major role in defending the body against disease.

Food is, of course, essential to life, although it is not always eaten in a form that can be readily used by the body. Most foods need to be broken down progressively, by the action of secretions and by physical and biological influences, thus reducing it so that it can cross the lining of the bowel and enter the vascular system.

Saliva not only lubricates the food but may contain an enzyme which helps in the breakdown of starch. The mechanical effects of chewing macerate food; the movement of the jaws also helps the release and mixing of saliva with the ingesta. In the stomach, the enzyme pepsin is involved in protein digestion and hydrochloric acid assists this and also the breakdown of fibrous materials. This process is further assisted by peristalsis, a type of gut movement that physically massages ingesta and moves them along; peristalsis is greatly assisted by the fibre content of the diet. Further digestive secretions are added by the pancreas, the gall-bladder and numerous glands in the lining of the bowel. While the horse does not have a gall-bladder *per se*, there is a continuous outflow of bile from the bile duct to aid digestion.

If we consider – in addition to what has been discussed already – microbial digestion, which is of considerable importance, particularly in the large bowel, we begin to see the complicated nature of the equine digestive system. We need, therefore, to understand it in depth, especially as the diversity of feeding practices today often challenges the simple working of the system as it is designed by nature. Failure to feed in an appropriate way can result in pressure on the tract leading to indigestion, inflammation of tissues and disease.

Finally, it should be appreciated by the reader that some aspects of digestive disease in equines are far too technical to be dealt with in a book such as this – which is essentially designed to provide a practical introduction to the subject for horse owners, those individuals engaged in the care and management of horses, and for the student. For those readers who wish for more advanced knowledge, the most appropriate sources can be found in specialist veterinary libraries.

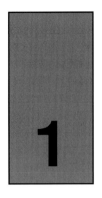

1 Anatomy of the Digestive System

The equine digestive system begins with the structures of the mouth, starting with the lips, the organs that first come in contact with food (for example, hay or grass). The food is chopped off by the incisor teeth, taken into the mouth cavity where it is crushed by the action of the molar (or cheek) teeth, lubricated by an inflow of saliva and eventually swallowed.

It can thus be seen that the anatomy of the mouth is complex, details of which are vital to an understanding of the part the mouth plays in digestion. The lips, while essential in drawing food in, also, through the action of muscles, form a seal that prevents the ingested food from falling out again while being chewed. The cheeks contain salivary glands but are also highly muscular in order to open and close the jaws in the process of chewing. As well as this, the cheeks enable the food to be kept within the area of the teeth, so that it can be crushed. This helps to break down the fibrous portions of the ingesta and allows the essential digestive elements of saliva, and subsequently gastric juice, to act on them. The tongue is an almost wholly muscular organ that moves the food about in the mouth and, when adequately chewed, propels it across the pharynx into the oesophagus. It also plays an integral part in the process that prevents any escape of liquid or solids into the trachea and lungs.

The Mouth

The first part of the digestive tract (also known as the alimentary canal) is, therefore, the mouth, or oral, cavity. It is bounded laterally by the cheeks, dorsally by the hard palate, ventrally by the lower jaw (consisting of the two mandibles joined by a sheet of muscle) and posteriorly by the

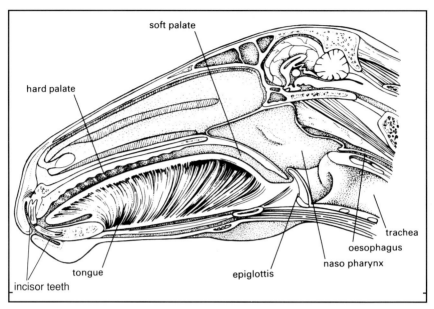

View of the horse's head in cross-section

soft palate. The entrance to the mouth, the anterior boundary when closed, is formed by the lips.

Inside, the mouth is arbitrarily divided into two parts by the teeth. First, the area between the teeth and the cheeks, the vestibule, is noticeable (especially in facial paralysis) when food collects and the cheeks become rounded by its presence. Second, the area enclosed by the teeth is the mouth cavity proper. When the teeth are in apposition, the mouth cavity is in potential communication with the vestibule through the interdental spaces between the molars and incisors on each side, and behind the last molars on each side.

The mouth is covered by a mucous membrane that meets the skin at the lips and continues over the tongue and onto the pharynx behind. The membrane is generally of a pink colour, but may contain areas of darker pigmentation. This pink colour is a significant indicator of health and it may alter to become pale in anaemia, yellow where there is jaundice; but it may also become temporarily discoloured by the nature and condition of the food being eaten.

The Lips

The horse's upper and lower lips meet at the corners of the mouth, the

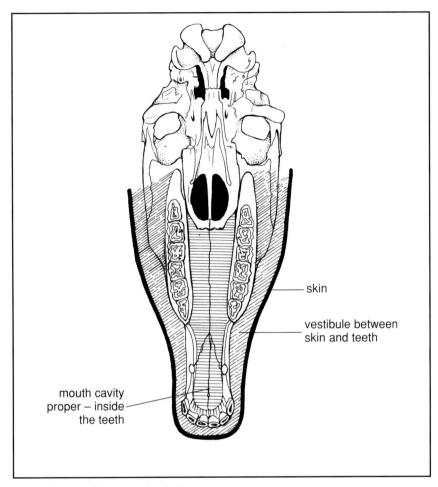

skin

vestibule between
skin and teeth

mouth cavity
proper – inside
the teeth

Ventral view of the horse's skull

commissures, near the first cheek tooth, and these junctions are well
rounded and contain the labial glands. As distinct from other grazing animals, the horse's lips actively grasp food and take it into the reach of the
teeth. Cattle and sheep, with only a lower row of sharp incisor teeth and
an immobile upper lip, make greater use of the tongue in prehension.

The lips are covered externally by skin containing long tactile hairs as
well as the normal fine hair. The pliable nature of the lips allows for a
considerable degree of movement, both for the prehension of food, for
swallowing water and other such needs. The lower lip continues onto the
prominence of the chin.

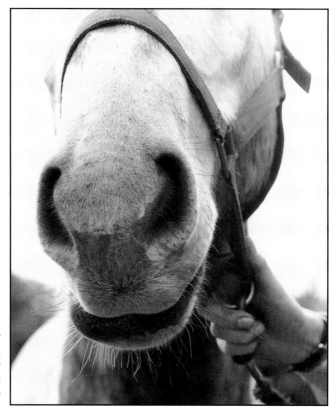

*Two views of the
horse's muzzle,
showing the
tactile hairs on
the lips*

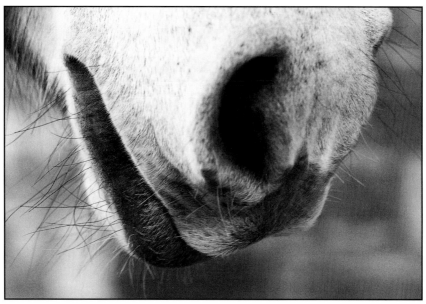

The mobility of the horse's lips, together with the tactile hairs and its well-developed olfactory organs, allows it greater freedom to pick and choose when grazing. The horse is a selective grazer. As is well documented, it will not readily eat from areas that have been soiled by urine or faeces. When eating hay, for example, horses will very often pick at individual pieces and deftly avoid that which they do not want. They achieve this mainly by use of the lips.

The Cheeks

Three layers make up the cheeks: the skin, a muscular layer, and mucous membrane on the inside. The skin in the cheek area is thin and pliable. There are two rows of salivary glands in the cheeks and the duct from the parotid gland usually opens on a level with the upper third cheek tooth.

The Gums

The areas immediately adjacent to the teeth are the gums, where the mucous membrane of the mouth is reflected onto the bony periosteum. It is this arrangement that holds the teeth in place.

The Hard Palate

Forming the roof of the mouth, the hard palate is continuous with the soft palate at the back. Its bony base is formed by the bones of the floor of the nasal cavity, namely the premaxilla, the maxilla and the palatine bones. The mucous membrane over the hard palate contains about 18 transverse ridges which are divided centrally, the purpose of which is to help guide the food back in the direction of the pharynx.

The Soft Palate

An extremely important structure in the horse, the soft palate is a common seat of breathing problems in the athletic animal.

Measuring about 15cm in length, the soft palate separates the mouth from the pharynx, except during swallowing, and slopes downwards and backwards from its connection with the hard palate. It is an oblique, valve-like curtain; the anterior (oral) surface looks downwards and forwards and is covered with mucous membrane continuous with that of the hard palate. Its posterior (pharyngeal) surface is covered by a mucous membrane that is continuous with that of the nasal passages.

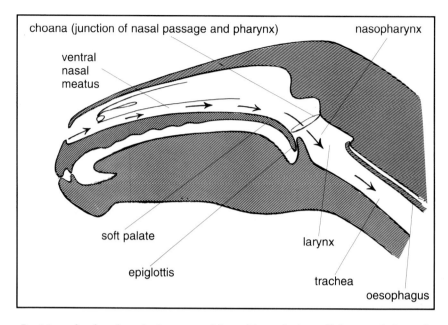

Position of soft palate during normal breathing, closing off the mouth from the air passage

Owing to its length – the free border of the soft palate contacts the epiglottis of the larynx – the pharynx is closed from the mouth except during the passage of food or drink to the oesophagus. The manner of this contact with the larynx is important, as a virtual seal is formed which especially protects the respiratory tract from aspiration of food material passing between the mouth and oesophagus (gullet) during swallowing. The large size and functional anatomy of the soft palate explains why mouth breathing is not natural to the horse. It also explains why vomited material (an uncommon phenomenon in the horse) usually escapes through the nostrils.

The Tongue

The floor of the mouth is covered by the tongue. The root of the tongue is attached to the body of the hyoid bone (a complex structure that resembles a child's swing, with the body of the hyoid bone being the seat and the sides being suspended from the underside of the skull) and to the soft palate and pharynx.

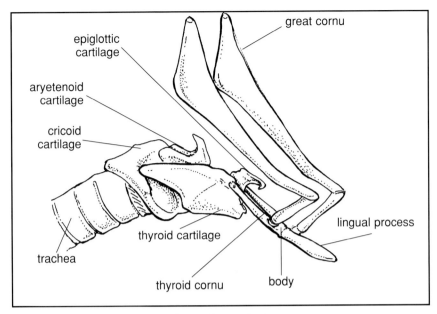

The hyoid apparatus and its relationship to the larynx

The body of the hyoid is also attached to the larynx. This hyoid bone is an important area of attachment for tongue, pharyngeal and laryngeal muscles, as well as serving to suspend the larynx in the ventral part of the throat. The hyoid is therefore critical to all aspects of movement in the region, both during eating and respiration.

The tip of the tongue, or apex, is free and spatula-shaped. It has an upper and lower surface and is rounded at its edges. The tip has free movement, as opposed to the root, which is restricted; a matter that becomes evident when the horse is licking an object. Unlike cattle and sheep, however, the horse does not use its tongue to grasp herbage and guide it into the mouth to be cut by a single row of very sharp incisors. Instead, the horse's lips, which are much more mobile, play an active part in prehension (though they may be drawn back when grazing) and the double row of crushing incisors cut the herbage as it comes between them.

The mucous membrane covering the tongue is particularly thick on the upper surface. This is partly due to the presence of papillae, of which there are four types: filiform, fungiform, vallate and foliate. The mucous membrane also contains numerous mucous glands. The purpose of the

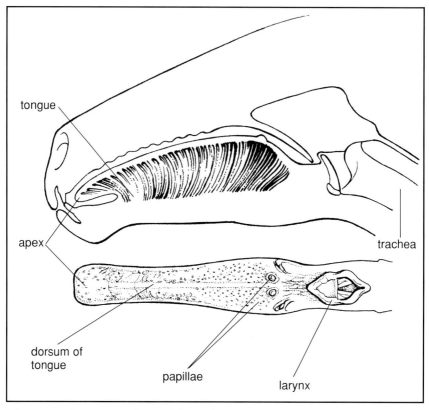

The tongue in cross-section and from above

papillae is to give strength and substance to the surface for the continual work it has to do. Filiform papillae are threadlike and scattered over the surface; fungiform papillae are larger and found on the dorsum and on the lateral parts of the tongue; vallate papillae are only two or three in number and found on the back of the dorsum; foliate papillae are rounded eminences found in front of the soft palate. The last three types are all furnished with taste buds.

From the lower surface of the free part of the tongue a fold of mucous membrane passes to the floor of the mouth – the *frenum linguae*.

The Teeth

Like all other animals, the horse has two sets of teeth during life. The first set of teeth are known as deciduous, temporary or milk, teeth. As the

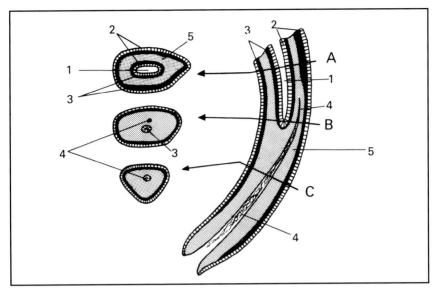

Incisor tooth in long section and in cross-section at the three levels, A, B and C. The shape of the tooth varies as it approaches the root. The structure of the tooth table changes in accordance with the stage of wear of the crown.

1=infunibulum; 2=cement; 3=enamel; 4=pulp cavity containing new dentine; and 5=dentine

animal matures, this first set is replaced by the second, and permanent, set of teeth.

A tooth consists of a crown and a root – distinguished by the fact that the crown is cased in enamel and the root in cement, a less shiny surface – both of which usually meet in the region of the gum. The greater part of the substance of a tooth is composed of dentine, and this contains a small central cavity, the pulp cavity. The infundibulum is a cavity in the biting surface of an incisor tooth.

There are four types of equine tooth: incisors, molars, canines (or tusks), and wolf teeth.

Incisors

There are six incisor teeth in both lower and upper jaws, and in both temporary and permanent sets. The wearing surface of each incisor has a depression in the centre (infundibulum, or mark) which disappears gradually with age. The shape of the incisors varies, being oval at the top and

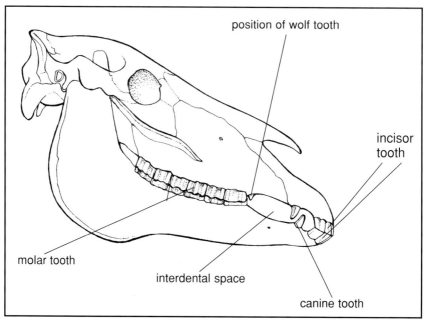

The skull, showing side view and position of teeth

gradually tapering to triangular at the root. Their purpose is to cut and chop food entering the mouth.

Molars

Large cheek teeth, with rough wearing surfaces, molars grind food. There are six molars on each side of either jaw in the adult animal – making 24 in all. These are described as three premolars in front and three molars behind. There are only three premolars in the milk teeth.

Canines (or tusks)

There is one canine tooth in each interdental space, top and bottom, between incisors and molars. They are usually only seen in the male. The lower pair are situated in front of the upper.

Wolf teeth

Not all horses have wolf teeth; in those that do, two wolf teeth appear just in front of the first molar of the upper jaw only. They are smaller than any other teeth and vary in size; some are little more than a pinhead and others are almost as big as a canine tooth. Because of their small size and shallow roots, wolf teeth are easily moved by the pressure of a bit. This

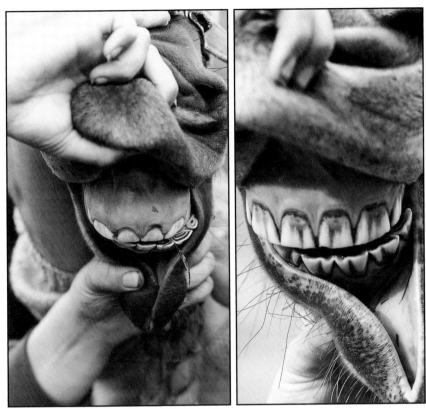

In a 2-year-old mouth (left) *there are six baby incisor teeth in each jaw, all in wear. In a 5-year-old mouth* (right) *there are six adult incisors in each jaw, but the corners of the teeth are not in full wear*

creates pain and may well cause an animal to throw its head about when ridden – often a reason for the removal of wolf teeth.

Teeth as indicators of age

Traditionally, the teeth have been used as a means of ageing horses. This has always been recognised as an imperfect exercise, although the reality is that many horses are capable of being fairly accurately aged, at least up to five or six years, when the lateral adult incisors have erupted and are in wear. Up to this time, the casting of milk teeth and their replacement by permanent teeth varies little. After five years, when all the incisors are permanent, it is necessary to rely on other signs for ageing (that is, angles, shape, marks, and so on).

Problems arise when it is necessary to accurately age horses for sale, or other, purposes, and when there is no documentary proof to support an opinion. At this time, variations from formally accepted guidelines may well make the exercise unsatisfactory.

In the adult horse the permanent set of teeth consists of three incisors, one canine, three premolars and three molars, on either side of each upper and lower jaw. The deciduous or milk teeth are smaller, the adult molars having no deciduous precursors.

At birth the foal has three cheek teeth – all temporary premolars, which later will be cast and replaced by permanent premolars – and the central incisor teeth. A 1-year-old has four cheek teeth, three premolars, the first permanent molar and a full complement of deciduous incisors. At an age of between 4- to 5-years-old the horse will have all six cheek teeth: the three permanent premolars and the three permanent molars. By this age, too, the deciduous incisors have been replaced by permanent teeth. The ages at which the incisors appear in each jaw are: centrals at $2^1/_2$-years-old; laterals at $3^1/_2$-years-old; corners at $4^1/_2$-years-old.

The corner incisor teeth are in wear at 5-years-old and are in full apposition by 6-years-old. At some five to six months of age the foal's wolf teeth may appear in front of the first premolar in the upper jaw. The tushes, or canine, teeth are usually present in the male, though small rudimentary tushes are quite common in mares. They appear at around $3^1/_2$- to 4-years-old and are fully developed at about $4^1/_2$- to 5-years-old, being generally absent in 2-year-olds.

From 5-years-old onwards, age may be determined by the shape of the masticatory surfaces of the incisor teeth and by the amount of wear as shown by the depth and appearance of the grooves which appear on their tables. Teeth wear down from crown to root; at the same time they are being pushed out of the alveolus (socket) by growth of the root. An outer enamel layer covers a layer of dentine and also lines the central depression (infundibulum). As wear takes place the enamel is presented on the tooth table in a definite pattern.

At 6-years-old, in a well-formed mouth, the upper and lower incisors meet in a straight line with no forward inclination. Later, they commence to incline forward until at around the age of 20-years-old they meet at an acute angle.

Notches (or hooks) make their appearance in the outer edges of the upper incisors at certain ages. For example, a notch appears at the posterior angle of the biting surface of the corner incisor at 7-years-old and, as a result, a projection develops at its posterior edge. The notch disappears soon after 8-years-old, and reappears at 11-years-old, to persist sometimes throughout life.

At 10-years old, Galvayne's groove, a longitudinal furrow often darkly stained, first appears at the outer portion of each upper corner incisor adjacent to the gum (in the centre of the tooth). By age 15 it has reached halfway down the tooth and, by age 20, attained its lower edge. Beyond the latter age the groove starts to disappear from above; it moves downwards at the same rate at which it made its appearance.

The Salivary Glands

Situated on the sides of the horse's face and the adjacent area of the upper neck, the salivary glands consist of the parotid, submaxillary and sublingual glands. As their name suggests, their function is the production of saliva, which enters the mouth through ducts, and helps to lubricate the food and assist in its digestion.

When the mouth is empty, saliva keeps the membranes moist. The flow of saliva is normally continuous, though the rate of production is

The salivary glands

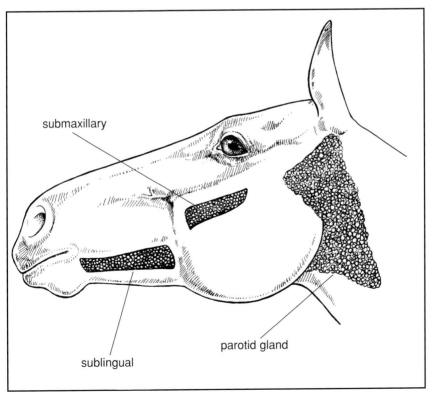

influenced by many factors. It is particularly noted in some horses that have just raced that the mouth is dry. This may be an expression of dehydration although some horses have dry mouths before racing, often attributed to anxiety or excitement. As Pavlov showed, the flow of saliva is naturally increased in the presence of food, and dribbling is often in evidence when animals anticipate being fed.

The Pharynx

A sac covered with mucous membrane continued from the mouth, the pharynx is common, in part, to both the respiratory and digestive tracts. It is divided into nasopharynx and oropharynx. The nasopharynx is the backward continuation of the horse's nasal passage, situated above the soft palate, allowing communication between the posterior nares and the larynx. The oropharynx is that area through which food passes from the mouth to the oesophagus, below the soft palate.

The purpose of the pharynx is to allow passage of food into the oesophagus from the mouth without interference with breathing and to allow air from the nasal passages to enter the larynx without any similar hindrance.

The division of these purposes is achieved by the soft palate, the epiglottis and the tongue. Under normal circumstances, when the horse is not swallowing, the soft palate almost surrounds the larynx, sitting beneath the epiglottis. When the horse swallows, the tongue presses back-

Anatomical openings of the pharynx

The pharynx has seven openings, not all of which are able to function at the same time, namely:

- Two openings to the posterior nares bringing inspired air into the nasopharynx and allowing the escape of expired air
- The opening into the larynx and trachea which continues the same process
- The opening to the mouth, which only opens during deglutition, at a time when the larynx is protected by the tongue and epiglottis
- The opening to the oesophagus. This is only open when food is passing through. The opening contains a sphincter (or valve) and is permanently closed except when forced open by the pressure created during the process of deglutition
- Two openings of the Eustachian tubes into the gutteral pouches on the lateral walls of the nasopharynx

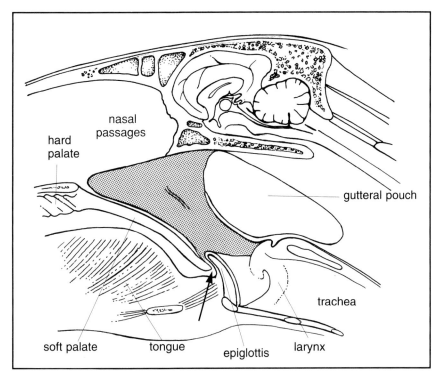

The extent of the nasopharynx (tinted area at centre) *with the soft palate* (arrowed) *beneath the epiglottis, the airway open*

wards, the epiglottis closes off the entrance to the larynx and the soft palate is moved dorsally so that food can enter the oesophagus and not be returned into the nasal passages. As soon as the food has crossed the pharynx the soft palate returns to close the seal and breathing resumes.

The pharyngeal wall is occupied by the diffuse tonsil, a structure which has particular importance as the site of entry of many organisms into the body – such as that which causes strangles (*Streptococcus equi*).

Swallowing is a voluntary act, after which all movement of ingesta is outside voluntary control.

The Oesophagus

An elongated tube that connects the pharynx with the stomach, the oesophagus is located under the skin in the jugular furrow on the left hand side of the neck before entering the chest cavity (the thorax). In the chest the oesophagus passes between the lungs and enters the abdomen at the hiatus oesophagus of the diaphragm, to almost immediately enter the stomach. Its position in the neck can often be seen when a food bolus passes along its length.

The length of the oesophagus is between 125–150cm, the cervical part (in the neck) being the longest segment. It is a strong, muscle-containing organ, capable of considerable expansion to accommodate boluses and is covered with a mucous membrane that lies in folds to obliterate the lumen except when food is passing through. The muscular coat is stronger at either end, especially so in the final third before joining the stomach, making gastric rupture more likely than vomiting in the horse. This effect is added to by sphincters situated at either end and it is the nature of the pharynx that causes vomited material to emerge through the nostrils rather than the mouth, when this occurs.

The Abdominal Cavity

Most organs of the digestive system from this point on are contained within the abdominal cavity (the rectum and part of the colon are within the pelvic cavity). It is important to appreciate the significance of this in the light of disease conditions that affect the different structures of the abdominal cavity.

Being the largest of the body cavities, the abdomen is separated from the thorax by the diaphragm, a thin muscular organ that plays a vital role in respiration. The relative size of the horse's abdomen is not fully appreciated externally because a substantial part is contained within the ribcage. Posteriorly, it meets the pelvic cavity at the pelvic brim, a line that is drawn by the anterior border of the sacrum and the front of the pubic bones. The consequence of this is that part of the ilia (the most anterior bones of the pelvis) on both sides help to form the walls of the abdominal cavity.

The lateral walls of the cavity are also formed by the oblique and transverse abdominal muscles, the abdominal tunic and parts of the last ribs which are behind the level of the diaphragm. The roof is formed by the upper part of the diaphragm and the bony and muscular structures of the lumbar area. The floor is formed by the *rectus abdominis* muscles, the aponeuroses of the oblique and transverse abdominal muscles and the abdominal tunic. It is the attachment of these structures to the xiphoid cartilage of the sternum in front and the pubic bones behind that gives the

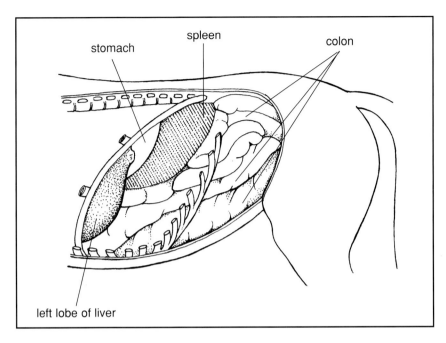

Outline of the horse's abdominal cavity: (above) *left lateral view;* (below) *right lateral view*

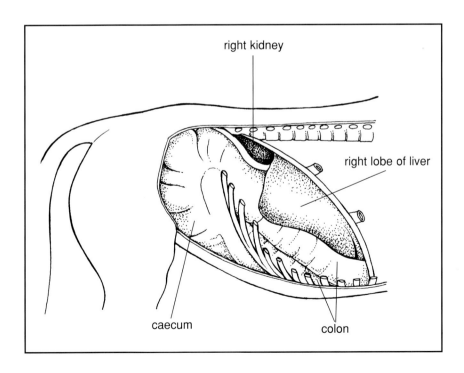

pelvic floor the strength to carry the weight of the contained organs, which may well include a foal in the case of the mare.

The muscular structures of the abdomen are all lined by fascia, a fibrous tissue layer that helps to bind muscle and add strength to related anatomical areas. Inside this, the peritoneum is a serous membrane lining the entire cavity and its contents. Besides the organs of the digestive system the abdominal cavity contains part of the urinary system, some of the reproductive system, the spleen, the adrenal glands, nerves, blood and lymph vessels and numerous lymph glands, all of which are intimately associated with the peritoneum.

The Peritoneum

A thin serous membrane (producing serous fluid) the peritoneum lines the abdominal cavity – and much of the pelvic cavity – and is reflected onto most of the contained organs. The peritoneal cavity exists between the two layers of peritoneum thus created, but it is a potential cavity, normally, as the layers are only separated by a light layer of serous fluid the purpose of which is to act as a lubricant, limiting friction during movement of the viscera.

The parietal peritoneum is that layer of the peritoneum lining the abdominal wall; the layer that coats the organs is the visceral peritoneum. Broadly, it can be suggested that the visceral peritoneum suspends the digestive tract from the abdominal roof as might a plastic pipe suspended in a sheet, the suspending sides adhering to each other when reflected off the pipe and held from an object above, such as a ceiling. The suspending sheet of peritoneum is called the mesentery (most correctly where it suspends the small intestine), the significance of which is seen in some types of colic. The peritoneum is also responsible for the formation of some ligaments within the abdomen connecting and supporting organs.

The pelvic cavity is, to all intents and purposes, the backward continuation of the abdomen, lined by the peritoneum in the greater part.

The Stomach

Situated behind the diaphragm and, partly, the liver the stomach lies at the front of the abdominal cavity, mostly to the left of the midline. It is a sac-like dilation of the digestive canal interposed between the oesophagus

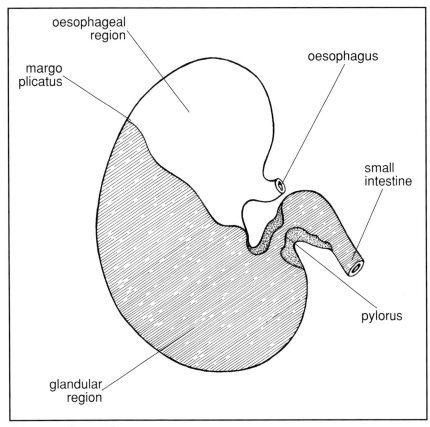

oesophageal region

margo plicatus

oesophagus

small intestine

pylorus

glandular region

Diagram of stomach

and small intestine and is strongly curved on itself so that the two openings, each protected by a sphincter, lie close together.

The stomach may be described as having two surfaces and two curvatures.

The opening into the oesophagus is called the cardia, this being closed by the cardiac sphincter, which is very strong and discourages reflux of digesting material from the stomach. The pylorus is the opening into the small intestine, seat of the pyloric sphincter, which lies just to the right of the midline.

The horse's stomach has a capacity of 8–15 litres and is designed to retain ingesta for a period during which they are mixed and subjected to the digestive influences of gastric juice. It is suspended in position by the pressure of surrounding viscera – and also by a number of peritoneal folds, the most notable of which is the omentum, that forms attachments between the stomach, the spleen, the liver and the colon.

The stomach (in common with the rest of the tract) has four coats: the serous (the outer), the muscular, the submucous, and mucous.

The mucous coat, or inner lining of the stomach, has two distinct parts, the oesophageal and the glandular parts both of which are readily distinguished in the opened stomach. The oesophageal part, which is off-white in colour and continued from the lining of the oesophagus, ends at a distinct line, the *margo plicatus*, which effectively divides the stomach into two halves. Beyond this line the lining has a different character, being covered by a mucoid, or sticky secretion becoming soft to the touch. This is the glandular part, containing the gastric glands and it is red in colour when fresh.

The Small Intestine

The continuation of the tract beyond the stomach, with which it is connected through the pylorus, the small intestine consists of the duodenum, jejunum and ileum. The small intestine is a significant organ of digestion and absorption. It is about 22m in length – the duodenum accounting for only 1m of this – and joins the large intestine at the caecum. The jejunum is about 25m long, the ileum being not much more than 50cm; the ileum being the final part of the small intestine that meets (with) the caecum.

The capacity of the small intestine is estimated in the region of about 40–50 litres.

The divisions between the parts of the samll intestine are not readily seen on superficial examination, except that the duodenum has connections to organs such as the liver, caecum, kidney and colon, whereas the rest of the small intestine is held (to the abdominal roof) only by mesentery. Microscopically, the differences are seen.

At a point some 12–15cm from the pylorus, the duct from the pancreas and the bile duct from the liver enter the duodenum. The diameter of this part of the bowel is about 7.5–10cm, whereas the average diameter of the jejunum and ileum is about 6–7cm.

The small intestine is generally held in coils within the abdomen, only the duodenum having a relatively fixed position in relation to the other viscera. The mesentery that suspends the small intestine contains vessels and nerves, also a series of mesenteric lymph glands and some fat. It varies in length from a few centimetres to as long as 50cm.

The wall of the small intestine contains the same four coats as the

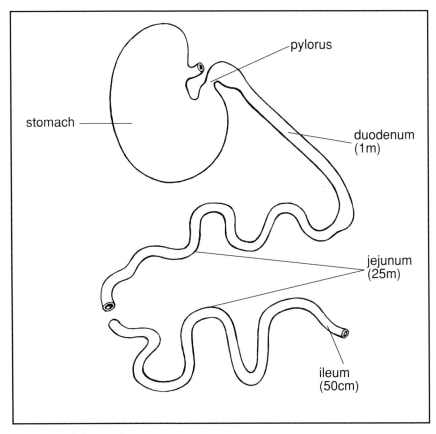

Diagram of the small intestine

stomach, and is most muscular in its terminal part, before folds of the mucosa project into the caecum to form the ileo-caecal valve. The inner surface contains numerous small villi, the purpose of which is to increase surface area. The glands contained in the submucous layer secrete *succus entericus*, the intestinal equivalent of gastric juice.

The Large Intestine

There are three distinct parts of the large intestine: caecum, colon, rectum. All are organs of considerable bulk, the function of which varies greatly from those already encountered.

The parts work together to produce a breakdown of cellulose in the

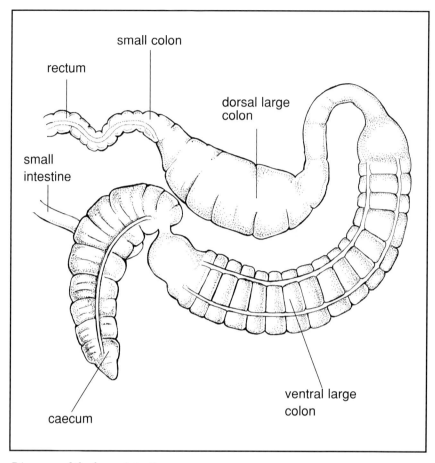

Diagram of the large intestine

digesta by bacterial fermentation, the absorption of these and other products (including water), and the eventual excretion of waste from the body.

The Caecum

The caecum is an elongated blind sac with a pointed apex. It is about 1m long and has a capacity in the region of 35 litres, indicating that it is a very bulky organ.

The body of the caecum lies in the right flank and tapers to the apex on the midline, on the floor of the abdomen behind the sternum in the fold of the large colon. In the caecum, the entry and exit valves are close

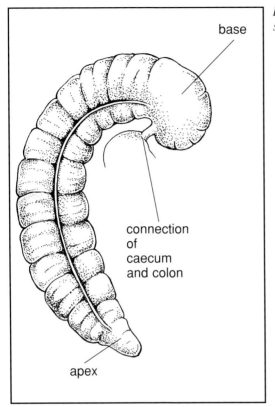

base

Diagram of caecum, showing folds

connection
of
caecum
and colon

apex

together, one to the ileum and one to the right ventral colon. A significant feature of this organ is the presence of four bands that give added strength and gather the shape of the walls into sacculations.

The Colon

The colon starts at the caecocolic orifice at the base of the caecum and is a voluminous organ. It begins with the ascending colon, about 4m long, and has a capacity in the region of 80 litres, being folded on itself to form a double loop consisting of the left and right ventral and left and right dorsal parts. Within these, the digesta pass along from right to left ventral and then from left to right dorsal. The first two segments have sacculations, like the caecum, the last two, having only a single band, do not. The right dorsal colon has the greatest diameter of the four parts, but it decreases markedly towards its termination to be continued as the transverse colon, which is situated beneath the roof of the abdomen in the region of the last thoracic vertebra, travelling from right to left. The descending, or small colon, is much narrower than the preceding parts, about 3m long and located in the left flank. This ends at the rectum, which is about 30cm in length and continues the small colon to the end of the alimentary tract at the anus. The rectum is contained within the pelvic cavity. It widens terminally before the anus into an area that stores faeces prior to evacuation.

The diameter of the large colon is as great as 50cm, whereas the small colon is 7–10cm across before meeting the rectum.

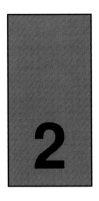

2 The Liver and Pancreas

Because of the complex part it plays in the body as a whole, and digestion in particular, the liver is of great importance. The pancreas, too, through the secretion of pancreatic fluid into the small intestine directly influences the digestive process. The roles of both organs are expanded on here.

The Liver

The liver weighs about 1.5 per cent of a horse's bodyweight; in a saddle horse, for example, about 5kg. Brown in colour, the liver is positioned against the diaphragm, under cover of the ribcage, and about two-thirds

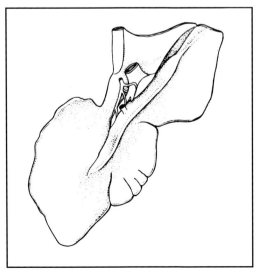

Liver of the horse: posterior view showing the main blood vessels

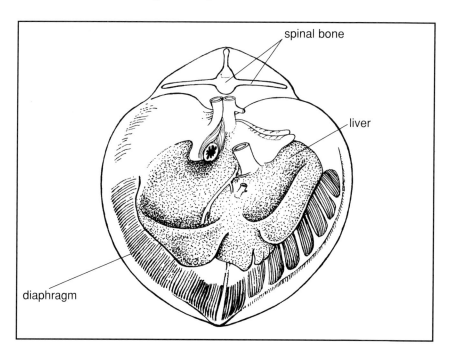

Diagram of (above) *liver with other organs removed; and* (below) *spleen, liver, pancreas and stomach lying against the diaphragm*

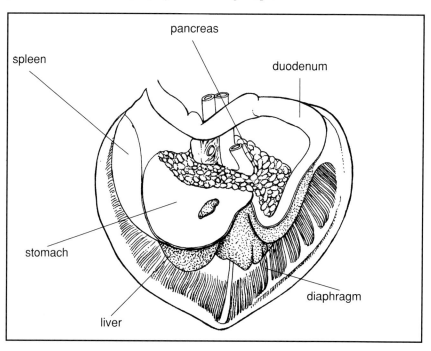

of its mass lies to the right of the midline. There are four lobes, and the horse's liver is peculiar in having no gall bladder. However, the bile duct is wide to compensate for this, and the nature of its entrance to the duodenum prevents the influx of ingesta into the duct.

The liver is one of the most important organs in the body. Without it, life cannot be sustained. It is a centre for a great deal of digestive processes as well as being a major organ of detoxification. Most of the products of digestion are brought straight to the liver in the hepatic portal system (of blood vessels) from the bowel. It also plays a vital part in defending the body against disease.

The blood leaving the liver is cleaned of toxins and foreign matter which may have entered the circulation from the bowel.

Schematic drawing of the circulation. Ingested material is taken to the liver before being used by the body

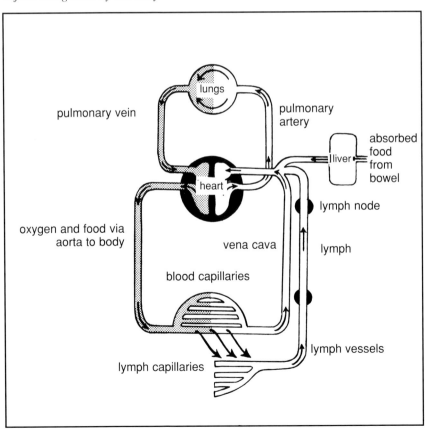

- Metabolism of protein, carbohydrate and fat
- Detoxification and removal of harmful substances
- Storage of vitamins (B12 and vitamin A), copper and iron
- Destruction of red cells
- Formation of blood proteins
- Secretion of bile
- Production of lymph
- Excretion of waste blood products

The major functions of the liver

The functions of the liver in relation to digestion are complex. By the production and secretion of bile, the liver directly affects the ingesta from the point where bile enters the small intestine. Elements contained in bile foster the breakdown of ingesta (most significantly fats) into finer elements which cross the lining of the bowel (by absorption) into the circulation. These elements are then taken to the liver where they may be subject to further metabolic processes before being incorporated into other body tissues as part of the process of life.

The liver is the largest gland in the body, its percentage weight being greatest in the young animal. It interacts with hormones to maintain stability within the body systems and respond to periods of metabolic stress such as hypoxia, exercise, overfeeding, starvation, and so on.

After an animal has eaten, the liver has to provide the immediate energy demands of the body, replace protein broken down in various tissues since the last meal, and maintain energy reserves within its own stores. The liver also has to convert excesses to immediate requirements (of carbohydrate, protein or fat) into triglyceride, enabling the excesses to be stored in fatty tissues about the body, including in muscle.

For the first two hours after a meal the liver is a net importer of nutrients; glucose, for example, being taken from the blood. Within four hours, ingested glucose can be depleted at which time liver and all other tissues begin calling on their glycogen reserves to provide energy. In a starvation situation, this demand can continue for about two days; production of ketone bodies (breakdown products of fat metabolism) during starvation reaches a peak at about three days but continues to rise for about two weeks. Modern practice considers that ketone bodies provide a ready replacement for glucose in starvation and that they are a readily diffusible fuel for muscles and brain tissue at this time.

The fasted animal shifts from carbohydrate and protein catabolism (breakdown) to fat catabolism. Fat can accumulate in the liver and excessive amounts are abnormal, which may lead to cirrhosis and impaired liver function. One type of fatty liver is caused by a deficiency of choline, seen in ponies. Pregnant, starving and lactating ponies are especially prone to fatty livers and the disease expression this can cause.

Clinical Disease Relating to the Liver

Because of its vital position within the body and the basic functions it serves, the liver is often involved in disease processes and any such involvement is expressed by symptoms which can generally be detected clinically. The implications are likely to be immediate as far as other body systems are concerned, although these may go unnoticed in sedentary animals. Whether this ultimately means a failure to cope with the demands of digestion, or to eliminate a dangerous poison from the body, the dangers are clear.

Causes

Liver disease occurs as a result of infection, poisoning (which may arise from sources within or outside the body), and abnormal metabolic processes (for example, fatty infiltration). The degree to which the organ can become compromised is substantial (60 per cent or more) before overt disease becomes evident. However, any degree of liver damage is likely to influence the athletic animal and may reduce the capacity to perform for purposes like racing, eventing, and so on. It may also have an influence on the development of secondary symptoms (like tying-up), and on resistance to infectious disease. The capacity to treat the problem will depend on the cause, and the extent of the damage, at a point when symptoms are recognised.

Leptospirosis is a bacterial disease that can affect the liver of horses, showing detectable jaundice. The infection is often associated with contamination by rat urine (in hunt kennels for example) and is also a regularly recognised condition of dogs. It can infect humans.

Of the viral diseases most likely to affect horses in the United Kingdom and Ireland, herpesvirus infection caused by EHV-1 is the most common. This may be mild and transient, and the degree of jaundice seen is variable, but the disease can be more insidious.

Equine viral arteritis can also cause jaundiced membranes. In the

United States, equine infectious anaemia is another possible cause of liver disease.

Ragwort (*Senecio jacobea*) is the most commonly met plant poison causing liver damage. Its presence can occur due to animals eating very small amounts of it, usually from sparse pastures. Its effects are often fatal. Ragwort can also be found in hay.

Tumours cause liver disease, but are uncommon. Abscesses occur rarely, but do have a potential to cause liver failure. Liver fluke is also a cause of liver disease.

Clinical Signs

Jaundice is a common sign of liver disease, occurring as a result of bilirubin appearing in detectable surface tissues. In human beings, skin may become typically yellow, but this is not inevitably seen in horses. However, jaundice is detectable in the membranes of the horse's mouth, nostril, eye, vagina or penis at an early stage. The degree of discoloration varies with the cause. Advanced jaundice with pronounced membrane discoloration is normally a sign of serious disease, with, perhaps, immediate implications for life; but lesser degrees of discoloration may well accompany reduced liver efficiency that might be very significant.

Bilirubin is a normal breakdown product of red blood cells, removed from the body in bile. Where jaundice is seen in surface membranes, the immediate concern is of damage to liver cells, but this could also occur as a sign of haemolytic anaemia, where there is excessive breakdown of red blood cells. Jaundice also results from obstruction of the bile duct, which in itself may be due to local inflammation or to the presence of parasites such as fluke.

It is important to appreciate that the presence of jaundice may reflect a secondary influence of disease outside the liver. It can occur as a feature of intestinal obstruction or where there is anorexia. Diagnosis of liver disease must therefore eliminate the possibility that such conditions exist.

Abdominal pain may be a feature of liver disease, although this would not be diagnostic on its own. Abnormal signs within the nervous system may be seen (for example, head-pressing, staggering, etc.) and any process for which the liver is responsible may be disrupted. This can lead to problems of blood clotting, leading to haemmorhage, or accumulations of fluid in dependent areas (oedema).

Laminitis may be a feature of some liver conditions and diarrhoea also. Discoloured urine is seen in liver disease, caused by the presence of either bile or blood pigments. Loss of condition is a common feature of chronic liver disease.

Cirrhosis, or hardening of the liver, is a consequence of chronic disease of the organ. It indicates a reduction of efficiency and also means that blood has greater difficulty passing through the liver, thus having implications for the vascular system.

Ammonia is produced in the intestine by bacterial and enzymatic action on ingested protein. It is taken to the liver where it is converted into protein. However, if this conversion process fails, ammonia enters the general circulation where it can become toxic. It also may affect other aspects of metabolism, resulting in lowered blood glucose levels (hypoglycaemia) leading to brain damage. Affected horses may show signs varying from depression to dementia. Yawning and incoordination are common signs.

Steatorrhoea is the presence of fat in faeces. This symptom can reflect diseases of the liver or pancreas.

Diagnosis

Clinical diagnosis of liver disease may be non-specific in the absence of gross symptoms. Especially if there is no marked jaundice, the only detectable symptom may be an increase or decrease in normal resting heart rate. Temperature may be normal, and membranes might show congestion, but this could also be seen in a number of other conditions, particularly infections, that have little necessary association with liver health or function. In these cases, it is necessary to have access to laboratory tests.

The presence in blood serum of enzymes which have leaked from damaged liver cells is a basis for the laboratory diagnosis of liver disease. However, such enzymes may also appear as a result of conditions that do not involve the liver and it is important in reading the information provided to take clinical signs into consideration as well.

Liver specific enzymes found in horses are sorbitol dehydrogenase (SDH), glutamate dehydrogenase (GLDH), and arginase (ARG), also gamma-glutamyltransferase (GGT). Enzymes present also in other tissues of the body as well as liver are aspartate aminotransferase (AST), lactate dehydrogenase (LDH), isocitrate dehydrogenase (ICD), and alkaline phosphatase (AP). Of these, SDH is a good indicator of hepatic necrosis in horses. LDH is not liver specific as it is also found in muscle. Occurring in heart and skeletal muscle as well as liver, AST is also released in haemolysis (destruction of red blood cells); increased levels after liver damage last longer than with SDH. In deciding that this enzyme is associated with liver disease it is important to eliminate other possible causes. For example, AP is not liver specific, although persistent high levels are a feature of liver disease. Persistent high levels of GGT occur in chronic liver disease, although levels may be only mildly elevated even in chronic cirrhosis.

Horses have higher normal serum bilirubin levels than other species. Abnormally high levels occur in haemolytic anaemia or anorexia, also in liver failure. An increase in bile acids in serum is a useful indicator of liver disease. However, high readings can exist without serious disease.

Blood glucose levels may be normal in mild liver disease, but low levels may be associated with nervous signs.

Low blood protein is not a persistent finding.

Prothrombin is produced by the liver and may be deficient in extensive liver disease or when inadequate bile reaches the intestine to permit vitamin K absorption. Prothrombin is involved in blood clotting, explaining why clotting failure is a problem in many cases of liver failure.

Bromsulphalein (BSP) excretion tests are useful in the assessment of liver function; normal clearance times for the drug being some two to four minutes; longer than five minutes is abnormal. For example, a 1gm dose is given to a 450kg horse by intravenous injection. Heparinised blood samples are taken before injection and every three to four minutes for 15 minutes. The time of collection is recorded and a graph made of the readings. Failure of the test to give a true indication may occur through perivascular injection, contamination of samples from the hands, improper recording, etc.

Further testing might involve liver biopsy, a technique that is useful where the condition of the removed segment represents the state of the whole organ. This may not apply where there are localised lesions, like tumours, abscesses, etc. Samples taken are submitted for microscopic examination and for bacterial culture where this is thought necessary.

Diagnostic ultrasound may be used in taking a biopsy, and may help decide whether the liver is enlarged, small, or of a normal size. Bile stones may be seen on scanning, as may cancerous growths, abscesses, haematomas and cysts. Radiography may expand on the information provided by scanning in certain conditions and the need for this will be decided by a vet. It is useful where there are dilated bile ducts.

Treatment

Oral, or intravenous, glucose sometimes produces dramatic changes in certain cases, but this may only be temporary. If given over a prolonged period, balanced electrolyte solutions should be added and blood and urine glucose levels checked.

Oral antibiotics can reduce production of toxins by gut bacteria, but can also destroy incumbent beneficial organisms. Cathartics (including mineral oil) may help prevent the absorption of toxins, or may assist in clearing toxic material from the bowel.

Electrolytes and glucose may be given orally, and it is important to ensure adequate water intake as fluid may be drawn into the bowel from body sources. Food quality is vital, especially dietary protein, making sure the food is both palatable and digestible to overcome a tendency to anorexia in liver disease. Good quality grass hay and grain diet is most suitable. Intolerance of protein is a bad sign, but may be expected and should be quickly dealt with by changing to a lower protein diet. Alfalfa hay has too high protein levels where there is a liver problem. B-complex vitamins are helpful by injection and fat-soluble vitamins also, though not essential. Vitamin K may be vital if clotting is affected. There is always a need to ensure that any substance given to an animal with liver disease is not likely to accentuate the problem. The provision of amino acids intravenously to horses with severe liver disease can have terminal consequences.

Specific Diseases Affecting the Liver

All the above symptoms are seen in generalised liver conditions varying from partial compromise to total liver failure. Signs of specific diseases that involve the liver may be different.

Photosensitization

The clinical signs of photosensitization, a condition marked by sensitivity to sunlight, are characterised by inflammation and necrosis of unpigmented (or lightly pigmented) skin, which may peel. The condition is distinguished from sunburn, photosensitization being a much more severe reaction that requires the presence of a photodynamic substance in the skin (a by-product of chlorophyll), derived from certain plants. A healthy liver is normally expected to remove this substance from the blood.

Signs of developing symptoms appear within moments of exposure to sunlight. St John's wort (*Hypericum perfoliatum*) and buckwheat (*Fagopyrum sagittatum*) are the most common sources of the substance; phenothiazine (a wormer) is another, though not often used now. The condition may also occur secondary to liver disease, when it assumes a more serious dimension.

The clinical condition varies from acute – with large denuded areas, intense irritation, scratching and self-mutilation – to a mild disease with only superficial irritation; but there are many grades of this problem seen. The areas of skin affected are those most exposed to the direct rays of the sun and the extent of the lesions will inevitably affect the outcome. There is initial erythema (redness) of the skin, with oedema (fluid accumulation) and pruritis (irritation). When the skin has sloughed (which may be extensive) there can be secondary bacterial infection, or invasion by blowfly.

The condition is treated according to symptoms, but affected horses are best taken into a dark stable away from direct sunlight. If there is liver disease, this must be taken into account and be catered for. Local lesions are helped to dry up by application of wound powder, or antibiotic ointments where secondary infections exist. The use of antihistamine injections may be effective in the early stages.

Serum Hepatitis (Thieler's Disease)

A condition which occurs in association with the use of serum of equine origin, serum hepatitis (or Thieler's disease) was first seen in South Africa. Immune serum was used in that country against African horse sickness, but the condition may occur with any biological product (for example, tetanus antiserum).

Some cases are thought to be caused by a blood-borne infectious agent, similar to human hepatitis B infection, though tests so far have proved negative. There is depression, yawning, ataxia (incoordination), headpressing, charging and coma. Marked jaundice is usual. Photosensitization and haemorrhage may occur, as also may haemoglobinuria (blood in the urine).

Diagnosis is based on clinical signs as well as laboratory results. The liver may have shrunken, and there is severe widespread damage to the organ. Some animals may recover, but symptoms may be very acute even though the development of liver pathology seems slow. Affected horses tend to recover or die in from five to seven days. A less severe, low-grade form of the disease is also seen.

Hyperlipaemia

A problem which may arise as a serious disease in small pony breeds, hyperlipaemia (excessive fat in the blood) is quite often precipitated by pregnancy, lactation or other stresses. In fasted ponies, the disease develops but then reverses when they are put back on full diets.

There is massive fatty infiltration of the liver and other body organs. Death follows convulsions and coma in about one week.

The signs associated with the disease are anorexia, depression, and staggering. Affected animals may be found standing over their water bowls, drooling. Diarrhoea has also been reported, as has ventral oedema.

Diagnosis is made from the symptoms and confirmed by the presence of fat in plasma (turning it a milky colour) and also high levels of serum triglyceride.

Affected animals should be kept free of stress (for example, transportation). A complete diet may have to be fed by stomach tube if the animal will not eat. Treatment is still speculative and aimed at dispersing the excess fat.

Donkeys may also suffer from this disease.

Tyzzer's Disease

A bacterial condition seen in nursing foals from one to eight weeks old, Tyzzer's disease (see Chapter 12) is often observed with evident jaundice and is caused by *Bacillus piliformis*. At post-mortem, the liver is swollen and has grey spots. The bacteria are seen, under microscopic examination, in the liver cells.

Tyzzer's disease is highly fatal, and any foal surviving more than 24 hours after infection will show marked jaundice and nervous symptoms.

Tumours

The presence of tumours in the liver is serious. They may be diagnosed on an ultrasound scan, and their presence in any horse is bound to have serious long-term implications. Such tumours are very often malignant.

Abscesses

Abscesses are most commonly caused by bacteria coming from the bowel.

Toxic Diseases

Pyrrolizidine alkaloid toxicity is a common cause of liver failure in horses and the poison occurs in various plants. Some examples of these plants are: *Senecio* (ragwort); *Heliotropium europium* (heliotrope); *Crotolaria* (rattlepods); *Amsinckia intermedia* (tarweed); and *Echium lycopsis* (Paterson's curse).

These plants are usually unpalatable and animals will only eat them where other feeds are unavailable. Some cases of poisoning occur after feeding contaminated hay, grain, silage and processed feeds. Spring cut alfalfa and alfalfa cubes are a common source. The toxic element appears to be in the seeds which may contaminate pasture or hay fields. Chemical analysis of the feed may be necessary to detect the cause, especially in cubed feeds like grass meal.

Symptoms may occur within weeks of exposure, but more chronic signs result from persistent low-level exposure, perhaps after a period of months.

The onset of clinical signs may be abrupt even though the condition has a chronic development. The main signs are central, like head-pressing, blindness, madness and staggering. Jaundice is almost inevitable and photosensitization occurs in a percentage of cases. Affected horses are in poor condition. There may be diarrhoea, ascites (fluid in the abdomen), anorexia. Abdominal pain may occur. Defective clotting may be evident and petechiae (pinpoint haemorrhages) on exposed membranes.

Liver biopsies confirm diagnosis, showing cirrhosis and bile duct proliferation. Advanced cases require destruction.

Ragwort poisoning is most likely to occur through feeding contaminated hay, as horses generally tend to avoid it when grazing. Death occurs in 4–6 weeks. There is depression, anorexia and the gradual development of jaundice. Nervous signs develop as the condition progresses.

Mycotoxicosis

Toxins caused by moulds and fungi can cause symptoms of acute liver disease. The most common of these are derived from *Penicillium* or *Aspergillus* species, producing such toxins as rubritoxin or aflatoxin on corn.

Aflatoxin (produced by *Aspergillus* species) poisoning causes acute liver failure in horses. Conditions required for production of the toxin are warmth and moisture: it is most commonly observed in tropical and subtropical countries, and is also known in the northern United States.

In horses, acute poisoning is most common, although a chronic form, represented by weight loss, lowered disease resistance and cancerous conditions, is also known.

Anorexia is an early sign of the acute condition and death may occur within 48 hours. Other signs include fever, increased heart and respiratory rate, and bloodstained faeces turning to diarrhoea with marked straining. Jaundice may or may not be a feature. In animals that survive the initial phase, clotting may be affected, with bleeding and anaemia evident. Ataxia and convulsions may be a feature. Post-mortem examination may reveal severe liver damage, haemorrhagic (bloody) enteritis, damage to the kidneys and petechiae distributed through the tissues.

Positive diagnosis depends on identifying aflatoxin in tissue or urine.

Treatment is wasted in acute cases. The source of the aflatoxin must be isolated and removed from the diet. Methionine is given to more chronic cases, also sodium thiosulphate. High-quality protein and fat-soluble vitamins are provided, also vitamin E and selenium where these may be deficient. Secondary bacterial diseases are treated actively due to reduced resistance.

Gall Stones

The presence of calculi (stones) in the common bile duct is named cholelithiasis, or gall stones. The stones vary in size from a few millimetres to as much as 12cm. They may be single or multiple in number and usually only occur in horses more than nine-years-old.

The stones are brown in pigment and contain mainly calcium and sodium salts, bile acids and bilirubin. It is possible that ascending infection from the bowel prepares the way for stones to develop.

Symptoms include pain, jaundice and fever and may be chronic with weight loss. The most common clinical sign is mild colic which may well be repetitive over a period of months or more, although a more acute disease syndrome may occur with liver failure. In this latter situation, colic, nervous signs and jaundice are seen intermittently, and there is frequently a raised temperature.

Serum enzymes, such as GGT, AP, AST and SDH are usually increased in this condition. Bilirubin levels are increased, as may be serum bile acids and serum fibrinogen. The clotting time may be delayed. These and other diagnostic results will be taken into account by the examining clinician.

On scanning, stones may be seen on the abdomen on the lower right side.

Treatment may involve surgery. Antibacterial therapy may be indicated using broad spectrum drugs, treatment being continued for several weeks. The prognosis is poor, whether or not a horse is operated on.

Horses with gall stones are best fed timothy hay, good corn and a source of B vitamins, such as brewer's yeast.

The Pancreas

The pancreas is positioned on the right side, beneath the abdominal roof, close to the duodenum and right kidney. It is roughly triangular in shape and lies close to the duodenum, into which the two pancreatic ducts open.

The pancreas is a gland, unusual in that it is both exocrine and endocrine in nature. It produces secretions (exocrine function) that are released into the intestine to aid digestion and also insulin, glucagon and other endocrine secretions, released into the blood, which are vital to the internal regulation of protein, carbohydrate and fat metabolism.

Diagram of pancreas in position in the abdomen

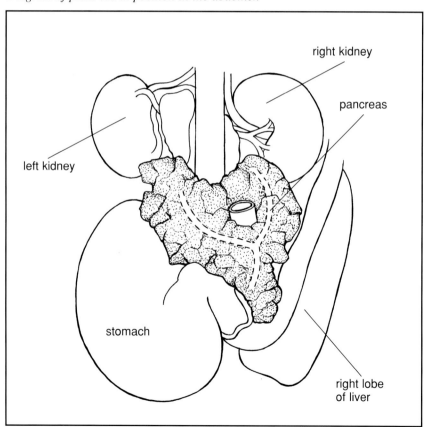

When a horse is at rest, pancreatic secretion is profuse and continuous, but the quantity of amylase (for breaking down starch) is relatively low. It provides a medium rich in chloride for ion exchange in the ileum, while making sufficient bicarbonate available to buffer fermentation products in the caecum.

Most enzymes are secreted from the pancreas in an inactive form (for example, trypsinogen) thus preventing autodigestion. These enzymes are activated by enterokinase or trypsin after entering the intestine. Additional protection is given by a mucus coating of pancreatic ducts. Plasma contains a number of enzyme inhibitors which neutralise enzyme that goes astray.

Clinical pancreatic disease is seldom recorded in the horse, due in most cases to problems of diagnosis. Hypocalcaemia (low blood calcium) is a common finding in acute and subacute pancreatitis. Pancreatic tumours are associated with chronic weight loss and digestive disturbances, including mild colic. These symptoms may be confused with hepatic disease, though there is seldom jaundice. There can be marked increases of liver-specific enzyme activity, which further confuses the issue.

Acute pancreatitis causes abdominal pain, progressive distension of the stomach and shock, often resulting in death. The cause is unknown. Migration of strongyle larvae takes them through the pancreas, causing inflammation of the organ.

Chronic pancreatitis is marked by weight loss, intermittent pain, jaundice and fever, with possible bouts of hypocalcaemic tetany. Mild liver and bile duct inflammation also tends to occur because there is a common papilla for the bile and pancreatic ducts in the duodenum. Fatty faeces are not seen in the horse, but there may be diabetes mellitus and a shortage of insulin.

Diabetes is a rare condition of equines, marked, when it occurs, by excessive thirst and excessive urination. This occurs because of disturbances in glucose metabolism, due to a deficiency of insulin, resulting in glucosuria (glucose in urine, which is diagnostic), and this provokes substantial water loss through the kidneys. The animal loses weight because of having to utilise body stores for energy production. The condition is progressive, but treatment with insulin has not proven straightforward to date. Insulin is also being used in some cases of hyperlipaemia, with varying degrees of success.

Atrophy of the pancreas can follow prolonged starvation. Most cases of pancreatic disease are diagnosed post-mortem.

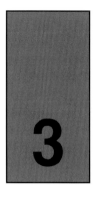

3 The Tract in Digestion

Digestion is a complex matter, and it is not the purpose of this book to explain the process in complicated detail, rather it is to provide a basic understanding that can be supplemented by further reading as required. However, it is important to appreciate the manner in which food is taken into the horse's body and how that food is dealt with so that it ultimately provides energy for activities such as racing and hacking as well as maintaining the horse's body framework and building new tissue. This chapter considers the part played by the digestive tract in this process.

Prehension

The horse takes up food by means of grasping it with lips and teeth and then cutting, or crushing, with the teeth. Water is drunk by suction, with the muzzle partially submerged, creating negative pressure through use of the muscles of inspiration.

Chewing is an important first step in digestion – and not just to crush and expose roughage to the influence of digestive juices – as it stimulates the production of saliva, which lubricates the food bolus for passage through the oesophagus and then influences acid-base balance on reaching the stomach.

The swallowing process entails, first, the gathering of a bolus of food material in the mouth. To achieve this there is marked action of the cheeks, crushing with the teeth, and pressing of the food against the hard palate with the tongue. As the formed bolus is forced backwards, the soft palate elevates and the tongue pushes it into the oropharynx.

The bolus is passed through the pharynx by peristalsis (a wave of

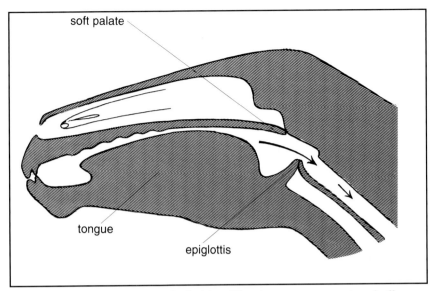

Position of soft palate during deglutition. The air passages are closed off

muscular contraction) created by the structures of that organ. There is a cessation of respiration and closure of the apertures of the nasopharynx by the soft palate. The larynx is protected by caudal tipping of the epiglottis, and contraction of muscles which draw the arytenoid cartilages and vocal folds together, constricting the glottis. During this process the larynx is drawn forward and upwards by the hyoid apparatus, the oesophageal sphincter opens to receive the bolus and closes immediately it passes through to prevent reflux.

Food is transported to the stomach by peristalsis, any failure of which results in regurgitation or, possibly, choke.

The gastric sphincter opens to receive the bolus when it arrives and closes immediately to prevent reflux from the stomach.

Saliva

Horses secrete some 10–12 litres of saliva per day. This fluid has little digestive enzyme activity but its mucus content enables it to function as an efficient lubricant preventing choke. There is also a substantial bicarbonate content, providing a buffering capacity in the stomach. Saliva also contains sodium and potassium, the concentration of bicarbonate and sodium chloride increasing during feeding. The buffering of digesta in the proximal area of the stomach is important, the balance achieved needs to be understood as the acidity, or alkalinity, of contents in different areas of the bowel is critical to the digestive processes. Any disturbance of this balance will inevitably lead to digestive upset and, ultimately, disease – perhaps expressed as local inflammation of the bowel and failure to digest food properly.

The flow of saliva is normally continuous, though the rate of production is influenced by many factors, the nature of food and amount of chewing required to break it up being among them.

- Saliva is produced by the parotid, submaxillary and sublingual salivary glands at a rate of 10–12 litres per day
- Mucus content lubricates food for passage to the stomach
- Bicarbonate content helps to buffer food in the stomach
- There is a continuous flow, which is increased during eating
- Saliva contains sodium, chloride and potassium

Summary chart: saliva

The Stomach

When compared with that of ruminants, the stomach of the adult horse is small comprising about 10 per cent of the size of the tract. In the suckling foal, it is relatively larger. Most digesta pass through the stomach in two to three hours, though the organ is seldom empty because the horse is a trickle feeder. When fresh food is ingested, stomach contents are passed on to the duodenum as new material arrives, a movement that stops as feeding ends.

A high proportion of water intake does not mix with food material in the stomach, instead passing straight through to enter the small intestine.

Some 10–30 litres of gastric juice is produced daily and this is stimulated by the presence of food in the stomach. Production continues at a reduced rate during fasting. The buffering capacity of saliva means the ingesta are relatively alkaline (pH 5.4) when first entering the stomach, and, due to the release of hydrochloric acid, this becomes increasingly acid (pH 2.6) as the pylorus is reached. Fermentation (the breakdown of carbohydrates to simpler compounds) occurs in different regions of the stomach, yielding lactic acid. The fall in pH towards the pylorus increases the proteolytic (protein breakdown) activity of pepsin (a digestive enzyme), though a relatively small amount of protein digestion occurs in the stomach of the horse.

- The stomach produces between 10–30 litres of gastric juice per day
- Contents are relatively alkaline in the oesophageal end
- Contents are acid in the pyloric end
- Fermentation of carbohydrates occurs in the stomach
- Protein digestion is limited
- Bacteria produce lactic, acetic, propionic and butyric acids
- The stomach contracts every 10–30 seconds

Summary chart: the stomach and its contents

Gastric Function

Masticated food, as we have seen, reaches the stomach with a high content of bicarbonate-rich saliva. Muscular contraction of the stomach wall then helps to further mix the ingesta. Liquid and small particle material pass quickly through to the small intestine, but heavier types of ingesta are held in layers.

The secretion of gastric juices is precipitated by the sight, smell or taste of food. Gastrin is a hormone released from pyloric glands as a result of the presence of certain food elements in the stomach (some amino acids, polypeptides, calcium, are examples). The release of gastrin is controlled by local pH – which, in turn, strongly stimulates the secretion of gastric acid and pepsin, having a subsequent effect on the secretion of pancreatic enzymes and bile flow.

Equine gastric fluid contains sodium, potassium and chloride ions as well as hydrogen ions. Acid concentrations in horses never reach the levels of animals like the dog, but sodium levels are high.

Gastric Motility

The horse's stomach has three muscular layers which influence the way food is moved through its lumen; contractions occur at a rate of about two to five per minute. The horse grazes in the natural state for the greater part of the day, thus ensuring a partly full stomach at most times.

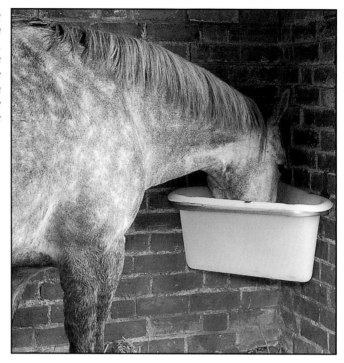

A horse eating from a feeding trough. Food enters and leaves the stomach throughout the process

The pyloric sphincter controls entry of food into the small intestine, but the stomach contents can increase considerably during feeding without adverse effects.

- Hydrochloric acid
- Pepsin
- Mucus (forms a vital barrier to digestion of the stomach wall by acid, loss of which may lead to ulcer formation)
- Serotonin (a hormone that inhibits gastric secretion)
- Gastrin

Stomach products

Pancreatic Fluid

The pancreas produces a clear, alkaline solution which is secreted in large quantities as a result of food being present in the stomach. This occurs through hormone activity as well as through nervous stimulation, peaking at 30 minutes after feeding and lasting for up to 12 hours. Stimulation of pancreatic juice secretion (and bile) also results from the presence of gastric acid in the duodenum. While secretion is normally continuous it increases four to five times when food is eaten. This fluid enters the duodenum, containing sodium, potassium, calcium, chloride and bicarbonate ions.

There is also a second element to pancreatic fluid, which comes in the way of a highly-concentrated enzyme-rich portion. This contains trypsin (enzyme that breaks protein into amino acids), lipase (enzyme for breaking down fats to fatty acids) and amylase (for breakdown of starch to simple sugars). The effectiveness of fat digestion here depends on the presence of bile salts for proper emulsification. The pancreas, as an alkali reservoir, helps preserve an optimal reaction in the intestine for the functioning of digestive enzymes operating there. Thus, food material leaving the stomach rapidly rises to over pH 7.0.

Secretin (a hormone), released from the mucosa when gastric acid enters the duodenum, stimulates the production of pancreatic juice, bile and intestinal secretion. Pancreozymin-cholecystokinin (PZ-CCK), another hormone, also initiates release of pancreatic secretions; gastrin assists this effect as well as promoting secretion of gastric acid.

During fasting, pancreatic secretion and enzyme production is greatly reduced, explaining why atrophy of the pancreas can follow prolonged starvation.

- Pancreatic fluid is produced in large volume
- The fluid is strongly alkaline in nature
- Food in the stomach and gastric acid in the duodenum stimulates fluid flow
- The fluid contains sodium, potassium, calcium, chloride and bicarbonate; also trypsin, lipase and amylase

---

Summary chart: pancreatic fluid

Bile

Mainly water, having only 2.5 per cent solutes, bile is a viscid greenish fluid, produced by liver cells. The main solutes are bile salts and bile pigments and small amounts of cholesterol, lecithin, electrolytes and proteins are also present. Bile is slightly alkaline in reaction. It provides a route for the excretion of many unwanted substances from blood while acting as an important digestive fluid.

The main bile acids are end products of cholesterol metabolism. Cholesterol is important as a structural component of tissue cells as well as being a precursor of steroid hormones. It can be synthesised by all body tissues, but more than 90 per cent is produced in the liver, intestine and skin. Bilirubin, the principle bile pigment, is mostly produced in the spleen and bone marrow as a result of the degradation of haemoglobin from old red blood cells.

- Bile carries waste from the blood
- It is a digestive fluid essential to fat digestion and absorption
- Bile flow is stimulated by the volume of blood passing through the liver as well as the presence of food in the bowel
- Bile is continuously released into the intestine
- Bile pigments colour faeces

The actions of bile

In the bowel, bile contributes to fat digestion and absorption. Bile pigments give the colour to faeces.

Disorders of bile formation lead to retention of bile pigments in the blood (and could be expressed by jaundice) as well as faulty fat digestion and fat absorption from the bowel. There may also be secretion of abnormal bile and the formation of gall stones.

Bile flow is also influenced by the hormone secretin. However, it is subject to other factors, such as the increased volume of blood going through the liver as food is being absorbed from the bowel.

- Inorganic electrolytes
- Bile acids
- Bilirubin
- Cholesterol and phospholipid
- Proteins
- Exogenous and endogenous detoxification products

Substances dissolved in bile

Intestinal Secretion

Mucosal glands in the wall of the small intestine produce the *succus entericus*, a dilute fluid containing water, electrolytes, mucus and cellular debris. Secretin and gastrin play a part in its secretion. To the medium thus being created within the small intestine (by the arrival of partially digested food) is inevitably added bile and pancreatic secretions, the constituents of which, including enzymes acting directly on specific constituents, play an important part in the continuing digestive processes.

Although the small intestine is long, digesta move quickly through and fresh food material may appear in the caecum as early as 45 minutes after a meal. Most travels through at a rate of 30cm per minute.

- Acid food material entering the small intestine is neutralised by pancreatic fluid
- Digestion here is mostly enzymic
- Mucosal glands produce the *succus entericus*
- Bile and pancreatic ducts are close together in the wall of the small intestine
- Peristalsis moves the food material along

Digestion in the small intestine

The Large Intestine

The walls of the large intestine contain only mucus-secreting glands which provide no digestive enzymes; peristaltic intestinal contractions move the digesta along. A large area is provided for the fermentation of digesta by micro-organisms and small amounts of water, bicarbonate, potassium and mucus are secreted by epithelial cells. There is a great deal of cellulose digestion and absorption of digested matter from this region.

Differences in the composition of food entering the large intestine occur with diet, but can be loosely categorised as fibrous residues, undigested starch and protein, micro-organisms and intestinal secretions.

Horses use organisms (bacteria and protozoa) to release energy contained in the structural carbohydrates of plants. The amount of bacterial cells in the gut numbers more than ten times all the tissue cells in the body. The large bowel produces no enzymes to break down cellulose, pectin and lignin into components suitable for absorption; but intestinal bacteria can do this, with the exception of lignin (present in wood, hulls and straw), meaning that foods containing high quantities of lignin are largely indigestible. This process is slow relative to the digestion of starch and protein; meaning also that digesta must spend more time in the large intestine to allow it to happen.

In ponies fed a diet of grain, one tenth of the food is voided as faeces after 24 hours, one half after 36 hours and virtually all by 72 hours. As most digesta reach the caecum and colon within three hours of feeding, it is the crossing of the large intestine that takes most time. Passage time is affected by the physical form of the diet – concentrates are faster than forage, fresh grass is faster than hay and so on. Food digestion time is therefore of critical significance to performance horses.

- Microbial digestion is of major importance in the large bowel
- Because of this, food takes longer to pass through
- There are only mucus-secreting glands in the large bowel wall
- Peristalsis is essential for moving the digesta along

Digestion in the large intestine

Gut Motility

In the small bowel both segmental (mixing) and peristaltic (propulsive) contractions occur. After eating, chyme (the mixture of partly digested food and associated juices that enter the duodenum from the stomach) causes distension of the bowel and stimulates local receptors; the receptors, in turn, stimulate motility in front of and inhibit motility behind the bolus, resulting in peristalsis.

The hormones gastrin and cholecystokinin increase small intestine motility, while secretin inhibits it.

Distension of one part of the bowel (for example, by gas accumulation in spasmodic colic) can cause ileus (failure of peristalsis) throughout the bowel. A rational approach to ileus in these cases is to relieve the distension, a matter that would be considered by an attending vet, if found necessary. However, that decision would depend on the animal's condition and many other factors.

Excessive intestinal motility may be provoked by bacterial toxins, moving ingesta along too quickly for normal digestion to take place. The consequence might be indigestion, or diarrhoea.

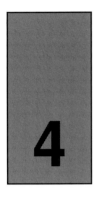

4 Digestion of Food

Digestion is the process by which food taken into the mouth is gradually broken down into constituent parts that are absorbed through the bowel wall and thus into the circulation. The process continues in the liver, but the degradation that occurs in the intestine is a fundamental aspect of the sequence of events. All activities, from growth to work, require the expenditure of energy derived from food through digestion. Also, as energy is expended, the heat that is vital to life is produced.

A diet of hay, oats and grass is composed of protein, carbohydrate, fat, water, minerals and vitamins. This food is digested in the various segments of the bowel, through the action of enzymes, organisms, and digestive juices which are released in large volume. The end products are absorbed through the bowel wall, the working size of which is maximised by the presence of villi, or finger-like projections of the lining membrane, that act to greatly increase surface area.

The diet also produces some essential elements (for example, certain vitamins) which are manufactured within the bowel by the action of organisms on the dietary constituents presented to them.

Protein

In simple terms, proteins are complex structures which are broken down into amino acids, partly in the stomach, but mostly in the small intestine, by the action of enzymes, before being absorbed. Protein is considered to be the 'building blocks' of the body, responsible for tissue regeneration, forming cell walls, membranes, muscle, enzymes, hormones, and blood proteins, and so on.

Protein is vital to growth, maintenance and repair and forms 80 per cent of body structure when fat and water are deducted. Its quality in the feed decides its value to the horse and this depends on digestibility as well as availability of essential amino acids. Studies have shown that the protein needs of adult horses are less when good quality protein is provided.

All proteins consist of long chains of amino acids. Ten of the different amino acids cannot be synthesised at all by the animal, or fast enough to satisfy demand for tissue growth, milk secretion, maintenance, etc. Plants and many organisms can synthesise all 25 amino acids; thus, the horse must have plant material in the diet, or products derived from plants, in order to meet demand.

The amount of protein consumed may be in excess of immediate requirements and although there is some capacity for storage by means of blood albumin, most excess amino acids are broken down in the liver with the formation of urea. Thus, an increase in blood urea noted in endurance horses may simply indicate tissue protein breakdown for conversion to glucose in glycogen depletion. However, it needs to be stressed that deriving energy from protein is an expensive and wasteful metabolic exercise.

- Proteins are the building blocks of the body
- Proteins consist of long chains of amino acids
- Essential amino acids must be present in the diet
- Feeding protein in excess of requirements may burden the liver
- A compromised liver may have difficulty dealing with dietary protein, or injected amino acids

---

Summary chart: proteins

Carbohydrate

Simple sugars (like glucose, for example) provide the immediate energy involved in all living processes and also ensure that the heat needs of the body are catered for. These sugars derive from carbohydrates (which are compounds formed from carbon, hydrogen and oxygen) and end up stored as glycogen for future use, or may be converted to fat (a reversible process) and stored in fatty deposits about the body.

Most non-structural carbohydrates (starch, maltose, sucrose) are absorbed before the food passes into the caecum; this would especially apply to a grain diet. Structural carbohydrates, on the other hand, are broken down by bacterial digestion in the large bowel before being absorbed.

Carbohydrate digestion and fermentation yields mostly glucose and acetic, propionic and butyric acids (volatile fatty acids). These nutrients are collected by the portal venous system draining the intestine and a proportion are removed from the blood as they pass through the liver. Both glucose and propionic acid contribute to liver starch (glycogen) reserves, and acetic acid and butyric acid bolster the fat pool and also constitute primary energy sources for many tissues.

- All activities of the body require energy
- Energy is provided by carbohydrate, fat and protein in the diet
- Carbohydrate is the most readily available source
- Fat is the means through which energy is stored in the body
- Protein is an expensive and wasteful source of energy
- In starvation, energy is provided from body stores, which may ultimately involve the breakdown of protein

---

Summary chart: energy production

Fats

Although fats can contribute to immediate demands for energy under aerobic (that is, in the presence of oxygen) conditions, they are, essentially, the body's means of storing energy.

Dietary fats may be digested and absorbed from the small intestine and later returned to the bowel and altered by bacteria of the large intestine. Bile salts help the emulsification of fat, following which lipase (an enzyme) hydrolyses these to fatty acids and glycerol.

Modern nutrition suggests the addition of dietary fat for the active horse has some benefit, and horses seem to accept this as long as the fat is not rancid and the level of fat added is not excessive. Investigations into the effects of feeding fats at levels varying from 0–20 per cent in Thoroughbreds have shown that the fats (fed as corn oil or soya bean oil) were efficiently used but the ideal percentage has yet to be decided.

Racehorses, and other performance horses, are sometimes fed additional fat as an energy source, one of the purposes being to increase energy density of the diet without increasing bulk.

Fatty deposits supply energy as the body calls for it, when either there are excessive demands or dietary intake is inadequate (for example, when horses are working, or in starvation).

As is commonly evident, the excessive build-up of fat is undesireable in athletic animals and there has to be a balance created between daily intake and likely demands of energy in these cases. The alternative is fat accumulation, with increased weight, and there is a loss of performance with other possible disease implications, like muscular injuries.

- Fats are stored in body depots from where they are recalled as need demands
- Fats can provide immediate energy under aerobic conditions
- Fat digestion is dependent on bile emulsification as well as enzymic and bacterial breakdown
- Excessive fat is a hindrance to athletic performance
- Excessive fat is found in a clinical condition of ponies

Summary chart: fats

Glucose

Healthy horses and ponies maintain a blood glucose concentration within defined limits. After a meal, blood glucose rises above normal resting levels (50–60mg/dl). Thoroughbred levels are higher (80mg/dl). Excess glucose not required to meet immediate energy demands may be converted to depot fat, or to liver or muscle glycogen. This process involves the hormone insulin, which responds to a rise in blood glucose.

Blood glucose reaches a peak about six to eight hours after a feed and there may be a return to resting levels in less than two hours from that point. Insulin prevents excess blood glucose from being lost in the urine by increasing the uptake in tissues and so lowering blood levels. In order to avoid hypoglycaemia (inadequate glucose in the blood) insulin is counterbalanced by other hormones (glucagon, glucocorticoids, epinephrine and norepinephrine), the system thus being kept in a state of dynamic equilibrium.

Exercise

In work, energy for muscular activity may be as much as 40 times that needed during rest. During a gallop, the horse's lung ventilation increases rapidly so that more oxygen is available for transport by the blood to the skeletal and cardiac muscles to foster the release of energy. This process cannot always keep pace with the demand and glucose is then broken down to lactic acid releasing energy in the absence of oxygen (anaerobic exercise). The fall in blood glucose stimulates the glucocorticoids (for example, cortisol and cortisone) and other hormones which enhance glycogen breakdown so that blood glucose can then rise again during moderate exercise.

The training process results in increased lung volume and, thus, capacity for gas exchange. There is an associated increase in red blood cells and haemoglobin to assist this. There is also a greater capacity for the oxidation of lactic acid and fatty acids to carbon dioxide. Training is associated with a decrease in insulin secretion, perhaps a higher glucocorticoid secretion, larger amounts of muscle glycogen and blood glucose and, consequent on the greater work capacity, higher blood lactic acid. The glucocorticoids, and possibly epinephrine, stimulate a more efficient breakdown and oxidation of body fat as a source of energy so conserving glycogen and yielding higher levels of free fatty acids in the blood. Glycerol released during fat breakdown tends to accumulate during hard exercise, possibly because of the raised concentration of blood lactic acid and only on the completion of hard work is it utilised for the regeneration of glucose.

The energy requirements of extended work can be accommodated by aerobic breakdown of glucose and by the oxidation of body fat, therefore accumulation of lactic acid is not observed in horses taking part in endurance events. Although body fat represents the primary source of energy, its slower breakdown means that there is a gradual exhaustion of muscle and liver glycogen associated with a continuous decline in blood glucose, despite elevated concentrations of free fatty acids in the blood. Exhaustion occurs when blood glucose reaches a lower than tolerable limit. In a more general sense, hypoglycaemia (inadequate blood glucose) contributes to a decrease in exercise tolerance.

Glucose represents a much larger energy substrate in horses given a high-grain diet, whereas volatile fatty acids will serve the same purpose in those subsisting on roughage. Horses on cereals will have higher peaks and lower troughs of blood glucose than those on roughage – due to insulin as well as the rate of consumption of the two diets. The grain-fed horse is more energetic at peak blood glucose and may be less so in the trough. The application of this is that grain-fed horses should be fed both frequently and regularly to keep blood glucose changes relatively stable.

Appetite

There is no established relationship between blood glucose, volatile fatty acid levels and appetite. A factor may be the amount of digesta in the intestine. Taste, visual contact between horses, energy density of feed, frequency of feeding – all influence appetite. It is also suggested that appetite is regulated by glucose in brain cells, by amino acids in the blood, by gastric and intestinal distension or contraction.

Urea Production

Urea is a principal end-product of protein metabolism, much of which is excreted through the kidneys. It is synthesised in the liver from amino acids present in excess of need so that a rise in dietary protein above requirements is associated with a rise in plasma urea.

While urea is within the tissues of a horse it cannot be degraded or otherwise utilised. It is a highly soluble, relatively innocuous compound and a reasonably high proportion of the urea produced in the liver is secreted into the ileum and conveyed to the large intestine where it may be degraded to ammonia by bacteria. Organisms containing the enzyme urease make this possible. Most of the ammonia thus produced is re-utilised by the intestinal bacteria in protein synthesis. Some, however, diffuses into the blood, where levels are maintained low by a healthy liver. If the production of ammonia exceeds the capacity of the liver and bacteria to use it, ammonia toxicity arises. Or, if there is liver failure, ammonia intoxication can occur without any increase in blood urea.

Microbial Digestion

Bacterial activity in the digestive tract aids in the breakdown of complex

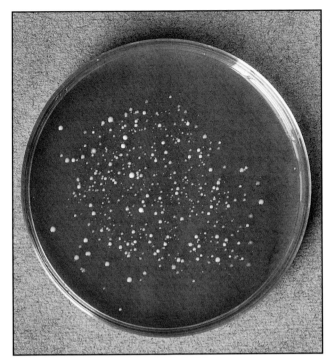

A plate of lactose-fermenting organisms

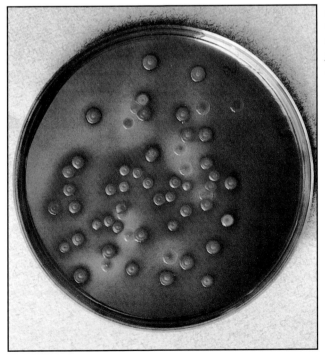

A mixed plate of coliforms and non-lactose-fermenting organisms

celluloses contained in fibrous foods. The degree to which this can be achieved depends on the amount of lignin present, which is indigestible to both bacteria and natural gut enzymes. Bacteria of the gut also synthesise essential amino acids as well as water-soluble vitamins of the B group and vitamin K.

In the fundic part of the stomach, which is more alkaline, 1,000 million bacteria per gram of ingesta usually exist. The species present are those that can withstand moderate acidity (for example, lactobacilli, streptococci, etc.).

In the large intestine, the bacterial populations are highest in the caecum and ventral colon and lowest in the terminal colon. About 20 per cent of bacteria in the large intestine can degrade protein, but the amount of protein digested there is only a fraction of that absorbed from the ileum. Protozoan organisms in the large intestine, which also play a part in digestion by breaking down starch (carbohydrates of plant origin), are far outnumbered by the bacterial population, but because of their larger size they contribute a similar mass to the total intestinal contents.

Numbers of specific organisms change up or down significantly during the day. These fluctuations reflect changes in the availability of nutrients (like starch and protein) and associated changes in pH of the medium. A change in the dietary ratio of cereal to hay will have significant effects on the numbers and influence the species present in the hind gut. Frequency of feeding can also have an impact on the likelihood of digestive disorders, reflecting direct influences on the bacterial and protozoal populations.

The microbial breakdown of protein, starch and fibre yields large quantities of short-chain volatile fatty acids, principally acetic, propionic and butyric acids, which could easily produce an environment unsuitable for microbial growth if not dealt with. This, however, is prevented by the absorption of fatty acids into the bloodstream and by the secretion of bicarbonate and phosphate buffers, which enter the large intestine from its wall and from the ileum. There is also the absorption of large amounts of water and electrolytes (for example, sodium, potassium, chloride and phosphate).

Caecal bacteria of horses adapted to a grain diet are less efficient in digesting hay than are the microbes of hay-adapted horses; and the reverse applies. If such a change is made abruptly, therefore, impaction, colic or laminitis may occur; and, when grain-fed horses have to adapt to a hay diet, puffy legs can be the result.

Microbial activity produces gases such as carbon dioxide, methane and small amounts of hydrogen. These gases may be absorbed, ejected, or take a part in further metabolism, and can be a source of severe burden when production rates exceed means of disposal.

A fine balance exists in the bowel because, in the absence of sufficient nitrogen, microbial growth cannot occur at a maximal rate and, therefore, a maximal rate of fibre breakdown will not occur.

Indigestion

Indigestion occurs when, for one reason or another, the breakdown and transfer of food constituents does not take place, or is impeded. From this it follows that a lack of saliva, for example, would not only fail to lubricate a bolus that might then fail to traverse the oesophagus, but the influence on stomach pH would mean increased acidity. Such an occurrence might well lead to inflammation of the lining, possible ulceration, and the food material that then rested in the stomach would not be digested in the manner intended. This material might then pass on to the duodenum in a state in which that organ is unable to deal with it, and so an unfortunate cycle of events is begun, with evident pathological implications for the horse. The consequences may lead to loss of energy, subsequently weight and, conceivably, later, death.

Symptoms may vary from constipation to diarrhoea, or may be so slight as to be ultimately responsible for, say, a mineral deficiency due to malabsorption. The example given relating to saliva is not likely to be a common one, although any horse that bolts its food is in danger. Stomach inflammation and ulcers are becoming a more frequent clinical finding nowadays and the cause for this has to be assimilated and understood by all those responsible for the care and management of horses.

In human nutrition practice it is suggested that the admixing of starch and protein as the main constituents of a meal causes problems for the stomach and can lead to pathological complications. Whether or not this has any implications for equine digestion is unclear. But it stands to reason that the nature of the diet, and the mix of food constituents, will dictate digestion time. And it is likely that food materials which are quickly digested are far less likely to complicate the health of bowel tissues than those that are not. Also, where combinations of food challenge the digestive capacity of the gut, and the organisms that assist with digestion, the same danger exists. Of course, the primary cause of indigestion might begin with feeding undigestible fibre, but it could also ensue from providing a complicated mixture, or by the addition of a constituent which the bacterial flora of the bowel was unable to deal with. It might also easily result from feeding foals at too young an age with food materials which their gut is unable to process.

Indigestion, as a clinical entity, is a common condition of horses. It most often is associated with the introduction of new materials into a feed and is a regular feature of early season problems in racehorses or competition horses, especially when they are fed poor hay. The symptoms are marked by performance problems. In most cases there is, too, excessive fermentation, with gas accumulation in the bowel and a surfeit of abdominal sounds when the horse is listened to with a stethoscope. In many of these cases, the faeces will be found to be unsatisfactory, either too sloppy, or too dry, and with much undigested material being passed.

The simple answer in this situation is to change the hay, an act that will usually bring the required result in days, if the replacement hay is of good quality. It is surprising how often this problem arises.

5 Ingredients of Food

Glucose is the characteristic sugar of blood and is produced from the breakdown of ingested carbohydrates, whether they be from sugars, starches or dietary fibre. Proteins constitute about 18 per cent of the horse's overall bodyweight and are essential constituents of all living cells. They are of animal and vegetable origin and are broken down to amino acids during the course of digestion. Fats are essentially the stored food reserves of the body, although they also play a more complex role in metabolism.

Vitamins are essential dietary constituents, involved in chemical processes which sustain life; some are included in the diet while others are subject to bacterial manufacture in the gut. Minerals are also vital to life and needed in constant supply. They are acquired from the diet directly. Trace elements are also minerals, required in smaller amounts.

The Living Horse

As we are aware, the horse is a muscular, mobile animal dependent to a great extent on its limbs. In the natural state, horses roamed the plains in herds, pursuing a natural diet, non-predatory, but subject to the advances of predators. They were constantly mobile, ever alert, even developing anatomical features that allowed them to sleep in the standing position. Their eyes developed in a position that gave maximum view of near and far dangers. Quick to move, explosive in flight, they developed great muscular power, innate athleticism, and bore offspring that were on their feet and part of the moving herd within a very short space of time.

The secret of horses' survival is strength and speed. It is these qualities

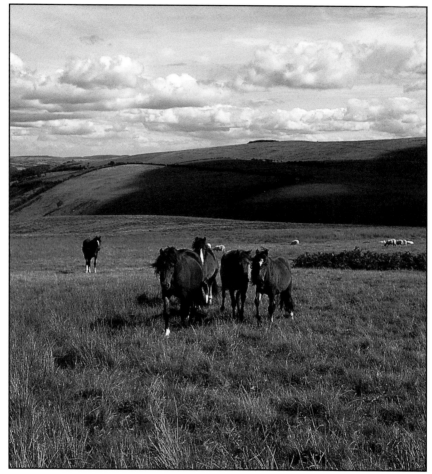

A herd of mountain ponies graze in their natural state

which today are the basis of most pursuits to which horses are put. The
musculature and the frame it is built on are the essence of equine movement. To sustain muscle does not require appreciable amounts of protein,
but the building of muscle does. The energy for work, be that jumping or
racing, is derived from the breakdown of carboyhdrates. Carbohydrate is
produced from the diet, also within the body by conversion from fats and,
if necessary, protein.

All essential food ingredients must be continually provided, otherwise
animals while able to perform will not be able to develop. When it is
appreciated that minerals such as calcium and phosphorus, essential in the
formation of bone, may be depleted by deficiency, the consequences are

easy to understand. And body reserves are soon depleted if they are not replenished.

Water

Water constitutes 65–75 per cent of the bodyweight of an adult horse and 75–80 per cent in foals. The horse needs water as a basis of life but also as a fluid medium for digestion, for milk production when required, and for growth. Ingested water also replaces losses that occur through the lungs, skin, faeces and urine under everyday circumstances. Total water loss occurs at about 20 per cent in urine, 50 per cent in faeces and 30 per cent through insensible loss. Restricted water intake will depress appetite.

Large amounts of heat are retained in water without a significant rise in body temperature. This is very important in the maintenance of body heat within acceptable levels. A rise in environmental temperatures of, say, 10°C will increase the water requirement by about 10 per cent. Work, too, depending on its severity, will raise water requirement by up to three times that of resting normal, and ambient temperatures and humidity will have a major influence on this requirement.

Peak lactation can increase needs to twice those of normal maintenance; a high-yielding mare may lose 12kg water daily in milk.

A great deal of water is lost through sweating – a process that is vital to body heat conservation. However, it is not adequate simply to provide water in replacement when there has been increased demand. Various electrolytes are lost in these processes and the body demands replacement to maintain fluid balance. There is a significant loss of sodium and potassium chloride in sweat. The horse disposes of excess salts of sodium and potassium and the breakdown products of nitrogen metabolism in its urine. With diets rich in salt or protein, more dietary water is needed to flush these excess products through the kidneys.

The average horse is said to have a daily water requirement in the region of 24 litres. There is likely to be a wide range of variation in this figure, depending on work, ambient temperature, and the nature of the diet. A horse in moderate training and kept indoors needs a water requirement of about 2–4 litres/kg of dry matter consumed, or 5 litres per 100kg bodyweight, per day.

In the digestive tract, water not only forms the basic medium through which most digestion occurs but also is vital to the absorption process. The quantities of water absorbed reduce as digesta move from the caecum to the small colon. The water content of small intestine digesta amounts to some 90 per cent, but the faeces of healthy horses contain only 60 per cent. The type of diet has a smaller effect on this than might be expected. Oats produce fairly dry faeces, bran produces moist faeces though they contain only 2–3 per cent more water.

The horse gets its water from three sources: drinking, water content of herbage, and metabolic water (produced as a result of metabolic processes within the body). Fresh young growing herbage is 75–80 per cent water, so consumption of it reduces overall body demand; but the opposite will apply in arid conditions. Most horses cannot tolerate water loss beyond 12–15 per cent bodyweight. Excessive consumption of cold water by hot horses may precipitate colic or founder.

Fibre

Dietary fibre is essential for stimulation of the bowel. However, where the quantity of fibre is too high, the animal is unable to obtain its energy requirements for work and the size and bulk of the bowel limit performance. It is for this reason that cereal grains are fed to horses in work, providing high levels of energy and protein per unit weight fed.

By reducing the amount of hay consumed, the extent of large bowel fermentation is controlled, and the physical bulk of the abdomen is notably smaller. While grass can, under ideal conditions, provide the horse with a great deal of its growth and energy requirements, the problem is that grass quality is a variable – in, for example, climates such as that of the British Isles. Nevertheless, horses are raced successfully from the field in many parts of the world, regardless of the limitations of grass, with the added support of controlled hard feeding.

Among other purposes, fibre is credited with increasing the water retention capacity of the bowel contents, affecting food transit time and helping to maintain the health and integrity of the lining membrane of the bowel. This latter point becomes important in weak or sick animals, where anorexia may result in atrophy of the bowel villi. Fibre plays a part in restoring these villi to normal size.

Lastly, where there is inadequate fibre in the diet, there is a tendency for the normal bacterial flora of the bowel to become unbalanced.

Minerals

The principal minerals are: calcium, phosphorus, magnesium, potassium,

sodium, chloride, copper, zinc, manganese, iron, fluorine, iodine, selenium, sulphur, molybdenum, and cobalt. Other minerals which occur in
tissues are aluminium, arsenic, barium, bromine, cadmium, chromium,
silicon and strontium.

This list is not in order of priority and by no means exhaustive. It only
goes to show the intimacy of our relationship with all the elements found
in nature.

Calcium (Ca) and Phosphorus (P)

The major structural elements of skeletal tissue are calcium and phosphorus. They are also vital components of blood. Substantial amounts are
found in bones and teeth where the body reserves of calcium and phosphorus are stored. Calcium is significant in blood clotting and also in
muscle contraction; phosphorus is fundamental to the formation of
adenosine triphosphate (ATP), occurring in all cells, forming a store of
high-energy phosphate bonds. During times of added demand, such as
pregnancy, lactation or deficiency, body reserves of calcium and phosphorus are called upon and mobilised. Both these minerals can be
absorbed into the system in the upper part of the small intestine, a process
assisted by the presence of vitamin D. However, phosphorus is mainly
absorbed from the colon.

The recommended dietary levels are 1:1 (Ca:P) for adults and 2:1
(Ca:P) for growing or lactating animals. Deficiencies of any of these substances, including vitamin D, can lead to rickets or similar conditions.
However, deficiencies also occur even when there are adequate amounts
in the diet, especially in problems associated with absorption.

Bone has a Ca:P ratio of 2:1, whereas the Ca:P ratio is 1.7:1 in the body
as a whole because of the phosphorus present in soft tissues. The elements of bone are in a continuous state of flux, growth and remodelling
proceeding continually. Blood calcium levels, however, have to be kept
within close limits at all times, otherwise serious disease symptoms may
appear.

The flux and distribution of calcium and phosphorus are regulated by
hormones (for example, parathormone) working antagonistically at the
blood-bone interface, the bowel wall and the kidney tubules. In the presence of vitamin D, parathormone maintains blood calcium levels by
mobilising calcium from bone. The kidneys of the horse play a greater
role in controlling blood calcium than does its intestine and this may have
a practical influence on disease.

Serum phosphorus levels vary without much effect (for example, strong exercise can reduce blood phosphorus to half). Bran disease, also called osteodystrophia fibrosa, is a diet-related disorder in which serum phosphorus is increased and serum calcium depressed slightly.

Failure of bone to mineralise is called rickets in young animals and osteomalacia in adults. In extreme cases, when calcium is being resorbed from bone for example, the outcome may be generalised osteodystrophia fibrosa. Here, fibrous tissue is substituted for hard bone and characteristic enlargement of the facial bone, and other bones, may occur.

A tendency to low blood calcium leads to increased calcium resorption from bone, increased excretion of phosphorus from the kidney, an increased rate of bone-mineral exchange, and a greater tendency of bones to fracture. Deposition of calcium salts in soft tissues, including the kidney, may occur.

Hypocalcaemia (low blood calcium) may occur after prolonged exercise (it is also sometimes seen in lactating mares) and is expressed as tetanic spasms, synchronous diaphragmatic flutter and possible collapse. The condition is potentially fatal. High temperatures may cause substantial losses of calcium in sweat which in turn may tax body resources and lead to tetany.

Excessive amounts of dietary calcium do not necessarily cause disease but may lead to brittle bones by increasing bone storage of calcium.

Calcium deficiencies may arise from diets low in calcium, or from grasses containing oxalates – for example, *Oxalis* (wood sorrel) – which prevent its availability. Diets rich in calcium produce a urine rich in calcium salts, and vice versa. In horses doing extended work, urinary losses of calcium decrease but sweat loss of calcium increases. Horses must absorb 2.5gm/Ca/100kg of bodyweight daily to balance the obligatory loss in work.

Calcium and phosphorus are generally absorbed from different parts of the gut. In the region of half the diet's calcium (and magnesium) are absorbed from the small intestine. Excess calcium can depress magnesium absorption, also manganese and iron, owing to competition at common absorption sites, or by the formation of insoluble salts. The site of phosphorus absorption varies with diet. No phosphorus is absorbed in the upper small intestine of horses being fed on roughage, but some is in those horses fed concentrates. The colon is the major site of absorption and reabsorption of phosphorus, a factor that is influenced by bacterial presence.

The nett available calcium in various feeds is about 50 per cent except where oxalates are present. The dietary level of phosphorus influences calcium absorption in that increased phosphorus levels inhibit calcium absorption by up to 50 per cent.

A mare may produce 2,000kg of milk in a lactation of five to six months and requires 10gm of calcium and 5.5gm of phosphorus daily to balance losses. This may be obtained from limestone or from dicalcium phosphate, which also meets the daily phosphorus demand.

- Calcium and phosphorus are vital to skeletal tissue formation and as elements of the blood
- Calcium is also associated with blood clotting and muscle contraction
- Phosphorus is an essential element of adenosine triphosphate (ATP)
- Body reserves of calcium and phosphorus are held in bones and teeth
- Absorption of calcium is from the small intestine
- The colon is the major site of phosporus absorption
- Calcium is lost in equine sweat
- Low blood calcium is a cause of tetany

Summary chart: calcium (Ca) and phosphorus (P)

Magnesium (Mg)

Up to 70 per cent of the amount of magnesium in a horse's body is found in soft tissue and bone. Magnesium is present in many enzyme systems, notably those associated with muscular contraction. Low blood levels can cause serious illness, although this is not common today. Muscle and nervous tissue depend for their functioning on a correct balance between calcium and magnesium.

An essential element of intercellular and intracellular fluids, magnesium is absorbed from the lower half of the small intestine, although some is lost through the gut and in urine. To replace this a daily maintenance allowance of 2gm/kg of diet is required. Magnesium deficiency is marked by nervousness, sweating, tremors, rapid breathing, convulsions, and heart and skeletal muscle degeneration.

Summary chart: magnesium (Mg)

- Magnesium is found in soft tissue and bone
- Magnesium is a part of many enzyme systems, especially those which are associated with muscle contraction
- Absorption of magnesium is from the small intestine
- Magnesium absorption can be depressed by phosphorus and by oxalates in the diet

---

In feed, the magnesium present is, normally, 50 per cent available. The most digestible sources are milk and lucerne. Large amounts of phosphorus in the diet depress magnesium absorption, also oxalates.

Potassium (K) and Sodium (Na)

Potassium plays a part in acid-base balance and also in osmotic pressure regulation. It is mainly found inside cells, where it has an important part in muscle contraction (its absence can lead to muscular paralysis). It plays a vital role in certain basic cellular enzyme reactions.

Sodium is involved in the regulation of osmotic pressure, in acid-base balance and in the transmission of nerve impulses.

Dietary deficiency of potassium may reduce appetite and depress growth. If a reduction in plasma potassium occurs, there may be clinical muscular dystrophy and stiffness of the joints. Spontaneous changes in serum potassium may result after strenuous exercise.

Foals require about 5gm/kg dietary potassium daily. Cereals are a poor source but hay contains adequate amounts. Thus, most diets should be adequate if there is at least a third of good roughage. Animals in heavy work consume more cereals thus lowering dietary potassium when losses in sweat would normally be increasing.

Diets containing 3gm/kg sodium are adequate except if there is excessive sweating in hot weather.

Lush pastures can contain large amounts of potassium in the dry matter. Although pasture grass may contain as much as 18 times more potassium than sodium, feeding supplementary sodium (in common salt) is unnecessary. Young foals may become deficient in potassium through persistent diarrhoea and this may precipitate acidosis.

Summary chart: potassium (K) and sodium (Na)

- Potassium is involved in acid-base balance, osmotic regulation, also cellular enzyme systems, especially those involving muscle contraction
- Sodium is involved in acid-base balance, osmotic regulation and nerve impulse transmission
- Hay is a good source of potassium
- Lush pasture contains adequate quantities of potassium and sodium
- Sodium is contained in common salt

Chronic sodium depletion results in tight skin, licking of foreign objects, inappetance, reduced water intake. In acute deficiency, horses lose coordination.

Chloride (Cl)

Closely related to sodium within the body, chloride is associated also with hydrogen as part of the acid present in the stomach and is an essential component of bile. Chloride plays a vital part in acid-base balance and osmotic regulation. As long as the requirement for common salt is met (that is, up to 10gm per kilogramme of diet), dietary chloride will be adequate. Major source of loss is sweat. Even at moderate work rates, horses may lose 100gm/day salt (60gm chloride).

While the use of chloride has not yet been adequately investigated for horses, symptoms of deficiency would include inappetance, muscular weakness, dehydration, constipation and, possibly, depraved appetite.

- Chloride is an essential ingredient of gastric acid
- Chloride is also a consituent of bile and plays a part in acid-base balance and osmotic regulation
- Considerable quantities are lost in sweat
- Chloride is also contained in common salt

Summary chart: chloride (Cl)

Trace Elements

Abnormalities in leg growth and development in foals and yearlings have been reported with dietary deficiencies of copper, manganese and selenium; and with excesses of iodine.

Copper (Cu)

A great deal of body copper is contained in the liver, where it plays an active role in enzyme systems. It interplays with dietary molybdenum. Copper is also active in the early formation of red blood cells, connective tissue, iron storage and the synthesis of melanin.

Copper deficiency is known in areas of the United Kingdom, sometimes due to excess molybdenum derived from underlying molybdenum rich strata (called 'teart' pastures). High levels of molybdenum and relatively low copper lead to copper-molybdenum ratios in the herbage less than 6:1, causing copper deficiency, which may also be due to low copper levels in the soil and herbage.

Symptoms ascribed to the condition are erosion of articular cartilage, anaemia and haemorrhage in pregnant mares. Thinning of the cortex of long bones may occur and fractures of long bones in foals.

A dietary intake of 15 mg/kg of copper is thought essential, although higher levels do not appear to cause harm.

The extent to which pasture plants extract trace metals from the soil depends on the soil pH and moisture content and the plant species.

Zinc (Zn)

In enzyme systems which function to aid carbon dioxide transport in the blood and its release into the lungs, zinc is a constituent.

Zinc deficiency depresses appetite and growth rate in young animals, causes skin lesions in adults and associated low zinc concentrations in the blood.

The dietary requirement of the horse for zinc is 50mg/kg and supplements used normally include zinc carbonate or sulphate. These inorganic salts possess a higher availability than do phytate salts of zinc in cereal grains and oilseed meals.

Zinc is one of the least toxic of the essential trace elements, except where there is industrial pollution of pasture. Toxic levels exceed 1,000mg/kg; a zinc dietary level of 5gm/kg causes anaemia, epiphyseal swelling, stiffness, lameness and breaks in the skin around the hoof. High dietary contents of zinc may lead to copper deficiency in horses.

Manganese (Mn)

A constituent of enzyme systems involved in carbohydrate and fat metabolism, manganese is also active in the formation of cartilage.

Manganese deficiency is thought to be a cause of enlarged hocks. Also, by affecting the growth plates, the effects of deficiency are thought to shorten legs and cause knuckling of joints. Excess limestone was reported in the United States to be a cause of high calcium in alfalfa and to precipitate flexural deformities. The latter can be corrected by use of manganese supplementation.

Young horses suffer lameness and incoordination when they lack manganese; and knuckling may occur in situations where pasture contains less than 20mg/kg dry matter of manganese. Severe deficiencies can cause foetal resorption or stillbirth and lesser deficiencies may cause irregular oestrus periods.

Iron (Fe)

A part of both the haemoglobin molecule responsible for the transport of oxygen in the blood and the myoglobin molecule, iron is contained in certain enzymes.

Iron deficiencies are unlikely, except where horses are anaemic through heavy parasite burdens. Most natural feeds are fairly rich in iron. The foal is born with an adequate store of liver iron and, from an early age, grazing will supplement its mare's milk (which contains meagre amounts of most trace elements).

Where iron deficiency exists the result is anaemia. A dietary concentration of iron up to 50mg/kg should be enough for growing foals; 40mg/kg is thought to be enough for adults.

Excessive quantities of iron are not thought to be toxic, although they may influence blood and liver zinc levels.

Fluorine (Fl)

As with calcium, phosphorus, and magnesium, fluorine is present in the crystalline structure of bones and teeth and so is an essential nutrient. In the horse the risk of excessive fluorine is greater than that of deficiency. Industrial contamination (especially from brickworks) of pasture causes weight loss and a softening and thickening of bone in grazing animals, but few cases are seen today. Dietary concentrations of fluorine should not exceed 50mg/kg.

A world shortage of digestible phosphorus has led to the use of rock phosphates in the diet, some of which are rich in fluorine.

Iodine (I2)

The formation of thyroid hormones, essential in growth, requires the presence of iodine, which can be the source of both deficiencies and excesses. Signs are similar in both cases.

Iodine is specifically required in the synthesis of thyroxine in the thyroid gland. Deficient pregnant mares may show no outward signs though oestrus cycles may be abnormal. Weak foals, with enlarged thyroid glands, may be produced and suffer high mortality. Certain grazing areas can be deficient in iodine and some plants contain substances that can cause goitre due to this. Enlarged thyroid glands are not uncommon in adult horses and, while some animals do not display any symptoms, others do not perform to expectation at work.

Dietary requirements are 0.4mg/kg of iodine. Excessive feeding of seaweed may cause toxicity, manifested in the foal by enlarged thyroid glands, leg weakness and high mortality in the first 24 hours of life. Foals affected in this manner may need milk from a source other than the dam; the milk may also be high in iodine, which will tend to further exacerbate the problem.

Selenium (Se)

Active in production of vitamin E, selenium forms an integral part of the enzyme known as glutathione peroxidase. Deficiencies of this enzyme in certain areas are an important factor in the condition called 'white muscle disease' in foals.

The importance here stems from being deficient. The requirement for selenium and vitamin E increases in the presence of polyunsaturated fatty acids (cod liver oil, linseed and corn oils, also pasture grass).

Selenium deficiency produces pale, weak muscles (both cardiac and skeletal) in foals and a yellowing of depot fat. Some foals are born dead or die shortly after birth. Those that live may have difficulty suckling and can experience respiratory distress.

Serum selenium levels may fall below 0.3mmol/litre in foals. In the United Kingdom, low levels have been associated with poor racing performance in Thoroughbreds (although there is not considered to be any association with the tying-up syndrome). Only in extreme cases is there muscle damage that can be detected by enzyme tests.

Selenium deficiency is thought to cause lowered resistance to infection and to be linked with reproductive diseases in mares.

Horses require 0.1mg/kg feed of available selenium. Plant selenium is the most common dietary source, although acute toxicity has occurred in sheep given very small amounts.

Some plants accumulate selenium (for example, milk vetch, woody aster, and goldenweed). Toxicity is more common in dry regions but horses avoid these plants given the choice. Where grass is sparse, animals suffer from 'alkali disease' in which excess selenium causes loss of hair on the mane and tail, lameness, bone lesions, deformities in foals and sloughing of hoofs.

Acute selenium poisoning is called 'blind staggers', and marked by head-pressing, sweating, abdominal pain, diarrhoea and increased heart and respiratory rates.

Sulphur (S)

Contained in certain amino acids (such as biotin, insulin, heparin, thiamin), sulphur is part of the building processes of some cells. Nutritional requirements for horses have not been established. Adequate, good quality dietary protein will usually provide for the sulphur demands of an adult horse.

Deficiency of sulphur has not been reported in horses. However, toxicity may occur by accidental over-feeding of flowers of sulphur, which is likely to result in death.

Molybdenum (Mo)

A number of enzyme systems incorporate molybdenum in their make-up.

It is known that excessive liming of land can cause a deficiency of molybdenum. Symptoms may include diarrhoea, poor condition, loss of hair pigment.

Cobalt (Co)

Vitamin B12 includes cobalt as a component. This vitamin is synthesised in the caecum and colon by the normal bowel flora.

The daily cobalt requirements of horses are not recorded, although horses do not seem impaired by grazing pastures known to be low in cobalt.

Vitamins

Vitamins are unrelated organic compounds which play an active role in metabolism. Some are contained in ingested food while others are synthesised in the animal's body from constituents that arrive in food. Organisms involved in digestion may play a part in this – for example, vitamin B12, known as the 'animal protein factor', is not available directly from vegetable sources, but is synthesised in the bowel by organisms.

There is little direct evidence of vitamin requirements for horses and most recommendations are based on those from other animals. Daily needs are met by the diet, by supplements and, in the case of vitamin K and the water soluble B vitamins, from microbial synthesis in the gut.

Tissue requirements are complicated by the synthesis of ascorbic acid from simple sugars in the horse's tissues, the production of vitamin D in the skin as a reaction to ultraviolet light, the tissue synthesis of niacin from the amino acid tryptophan and the partial substitution of a need for choline by methionine and other sources of methyl groups.

Dietary needs for vitamin D increase when animals are kept indoors, away from direct sunlight, have thick coats, or highly pigmented skin, and so on.

Foals have a higher requirement for B vitamins and vitamin K because of the immaturity of the gut. Lactating mares will also have a higher requirement for vitamins than will barren mares, but this may be balanced by increased appetite. A good grazing season on high-quality grass can satisfy the mare's winter need for vitamin A. But there may be a decline in digestive efficiency with age, possibly linked with parasites as well as infectious diseases of the bowel.

Essential Sources

For herbivorous animals, grass can provide all the necessary ingredients of a balanced diet. However, bulk is a problem for competing horses, because of the need to curtail large bowel fermentation, thus necessitating the use of concentrates. Also, grass is seasonal, varying in quality as the growing year advances, and unsuitable to systems of management where horses spend most of their time stabled.

The problem of grass bulk is partly solved by drying, but in the process vitamin values are reduced. Further reduction is caused by bad harvesting, as vitamins are adversely affected by excessive heat and fermentation as well as by too much sun. Kiln drying of grain can also affect vitamin content.

Where a diet contains good hay, cut young so the seed is not lost, oats, bran and carrots, an ample supply of most vitamins will be present. Reputable feed compounders are careful that their products cater for the same need anyway. However, there are innumerable feed supplements available as well.

For young growing animals the need for balanced intake of essential vitamins and minerals cannot be over-stressed. Deficiencies will occur when there is any shortage; the most common of these are ricket-type conditions associated with bone development. This deficiency must not be confused with enlargements of the epiphyseal plates in foals due to concussion on hard ground – mostly noted on fetlock joints. In this case, the animal will grow into the leg and the enlargements will disappear in time. However, it is very important in both situations to assess diet and ensure there is no imbalance of calcium and phosphorus and of adequate vitamins A, D, and E.

Foals fed on oats and bran need a balanced intake of calcium and phosphorus. Bran is a rich source of phosphorus and when fed alone can cause disease in horses of any age. Where foals are fed on grain it is necessary to ensure vitamins and minerals are being provided.

It should be mentioned here that excessive supplies of vitamins are unnecessary and may be harmful. Specific symptoms result from vitamin deficiencies and from excesses. Just as foals kept in dark stables may be short of vitamin D – the sunshine vitamin – feeding excessive amounts of the same vitamin causes toxicity.

Even when the B vitamin complex is available from normal food sources, including gut synthesis, deficiencies may still occur where there is added demand – as in the racehorse, for example. It is important, therefore, that supplements be available where needed in such situations.

Fat-soluble Vitamins

Vitamins A, D, E and K are the fat-soluble vitamins. Any disease condition affecting fat absorption will also affect the absorption of these vitamins, a situation that has also been blamed on dosing with mineral oil.

Vitamin A (Retinol)

The formation of bone and development of vision are influenced by the levels of vitamin A in the body. The levels, too, affect the health of cells lining body structures and are therefore reflected in disease resistance.

Vitamin A is essential for normal development in the young and in reproduction. The vitamin is of animal origin, though many precursors are available from grass and vegetables such as carrots. Feeding too much vitamin A can cause toxicity. Large amounts of the precursor are lost in the curing and storage of hay.

Grazing horses derive their vitamin A from the carotenoid pigments present in herbage. Fresh leafy herbage contains the equivalent of some 100,000–200,000 IU vitamin A per kilogramme of dry matter. Hay that is not green contains virtually no vitamin A. Good pasture normally would provide sufficient daily intake.

Signs of vitamin A deficiency are excessive lacrimation, poor bone development, faulty night vision, scaling and thickening of the skin, and increased respiratory infection. It could be associated with poor fertility in the mare. These signs are rare and only occur in extreme conditions of deprivation. Stabled horses need positive sources of this vitamin.

A daily intake of 50,000 IU vitamin A is sufficient for all horses and a dosage of ten times that may be toxic. Synthetic forms of vitamin A are stabilised and retain their potency for several years. Deficiencies occur through failure to supplement feed or by providing badly-stored feed.

Vitamin A deficiency may occur in horses fed only on poor quality hay. Signs of excess levels are unusual and are unlikely to occur under natural conditions. Bone fragility is one suggested effect.

Vitamin D (Calciferol)

Absorption of calcium and phosphorus from the intestine is facilitated by vitamin D and it also assists in the formation of bone. It is found in hay and is synthesised in the skin on exposure to sunlight. Fish oils are a rich source. Absence of sunlight may cause a deficiency.

Under the influence of parathormone (secreted by the parathyroid gland), vitamin D is converted to its active form, a steroid hormone in the kidney. This hormone has two targets, the small intestine and bone. In the small intestine, it stimulates the absorption of calcium and phosphorus from the ingesta. In bone, it mobilises bone minerals. In the kidney tubules, parathormone stimulates the reabsorption of calcium but blocks the reabsorption of phosphorus. The objective of the two hormones, together with thyrocalcitonin, is to sustain blood calcium levels. When the diet is deficient in calcium but adequate in phosphorus, a fall in plasma calcium ions triggers the release of parathormone. This stimulates renal calcium reabsorption and the production of the vitamin D hormone. Intestinal absorption and bone mobilisation of calcium is facilitated so that blood calcium levels are returned to normal.

In the absence of vitamin D, absorption of calcium from the bowel and release of calcium from bone are both depressed, thus blood calcium levels fall. Some mobilisation of bone calcium continues, so that osteomalacia (decalcification) occurs in adult horses and rickets (reduced calcification) in the young. There is loss of appetite, discomfort, lameness, increased risk of fractures and thinning of long bone. In young horses the epiphyses are enlarged and late in closing.

An adequate daily food intake is 1,000 IU of Vitamin D per kilogramme. Excessive amounts will cause signs similar to deficiency and eventual death, due to the effect of the vitamin D hormone on bone mineral mobilisation. Some plant species synthesise this active hormone and so can lead to rickets and soft-tissue calcification; in the United States, for example, wild jasmine, a member of the potato family, produces the hormone in Florida, Texas and California.

Vitamin E (Alpha-tocopherol)

Vitamin E is a factor in reproduction, but it also plays a major part in the integrity of the muscular system. It is interrelated with selenium, with which it helps to prevent muscular dystrophy. Cereal grains, green plants and hay are good sources.

Although vitamin E has a property that protects other substances in food from oxidation, it is itself capable of being destroyed by oxidation. This is accelerated by poor storage, by mould damage, by ensilage or by preserving cereals in moist conditions. After the crushing of oats or the grinding of cereals, vitamin E is gradually destroyed unless the material is pelleted. Fresh, green forage and the germ of cereal grains are rich sources of vitamin E. Modern feeds are frequently supplemented with a stable form of the vitamin.

The horse stores vitamin E less well than it does vitamin A and the onset of deficiency is accelerated when the diet contains insufficient selenium and is rich in unsaturated fats. Vitamin E acts by protecting unsaturated lipids in tissue from oxidation. In conditions where the intake of selenium and vitamin E is low, which may occur on pasture, mares can give birth to foals suffering from muscle degeneration. These foals may be born dead or die soon after; the damage to the muscles is thought to be irreversible.

The use of vitamin E and selenium in tying-up is commonly mentioned, but unproven. It has to be appreciated that this condition arises from a complex of reasons and, in treating it, the underlying cause must be found so that it can be reversed. Furthermore, deficiencies of vitamin E are not a problem in animals fed balanced diets, and supplementation is often surplus to requirements. There is also a suggestion that supplementary vitamin E helps fertility in mares and stallions, though deficiencies are only likely to occur in animals on inadequate diets.

Although more vitamin E may be needed when selenium is deficient, both are required nutrients and the amount of vitamin E that should be present in the diet rises in proportion to the level of dietary unsaturated fats. Suggested daily intake is 4mg/kg bodyweight. Rations for horses should contain 75 IU vitamin E per kilogramme. Foals may need more and idle adult horses less.

Vitamin K

In the clotting mechanism of blood, vitamin K plays an important part. It is generally synthesised in the intestine of animals, but hay and pasture are rich sources. Vitamin K, along with the B vitamins, is synthesised by gut organisms in amounts that should normally meet the horse's daily needs. This may not be adequate in the first weeks of life or where there is prolonged sulphonamide treatment.

Although vitamin K is essential for clotting, it is not related to respiratory bleeding in racehorses, which is thought to be due to a combination of on-going lung pathology and blood vessel fragility. There is some body storage of vitamin K and natural feeds, particularly leafy material, are fairly rich sources so that no supplementation is needed.

Water-soluble Vitamins

Normal intestinal synthesis plus amounts present in standard horse feeds seem to meet the maintenance requirements for riboflavin, nicotinic acid, pantothenic acid, and pyridoxine. If there is a change in diet towards root vegetables and by-products, supplementation may be needed. The needs of lactating mares and weanling foals are met by good quality pasture.

Thiamin (vitamin B1)

Thiamin is closely involved in cell metabolism. Brewer's yeast is a very good source, as are cereal grains and hay. Deficiency causes anorexia, incoordination, dilation and hypertrophy of the heart; also a decline in blood thiamin and the activity of enzymes using thiamin as a co-factor.

Bracken poisoning causes thiamin deficiency.

A total dietary level of 3mg/kg feed would appear to meet thiamin requirements. It is not known if there is an increasing demand with exercise. Thiamin given in single doses of 1,000-2,000mg is said to have a marked sedative effect on nervous racehorses.

Vitamin B12 (cyanocobalamin)

Known as the 'anti-pernicious-anaemia factor', showing its part in blood metabolism, vitamin B12 is not contained in any vegetable source and is synthesised by organisms in the gut of the horse. However, although deficiencies are said to be unlikely in practice, supplementation is sometimes seen to have significant effect.

The cyanocobalamin molecule contains cobalt. Horses appear to have low requirements for cobalt but require about 0.1mg/kg diet for adequate intestinal synthesis of vitamin B12. The vitamin is used in red cell replication and deficiencies are associated with anaemia. Adult horses in training on high-grain rations may need supplementation because a decline in appetite may reflect a build up of blood propionate. This volatile fatty acid is produced in greater quantity in these circumstances and its metabolism to succinate depends on an enzyme that uses cyanocobalamin as a co-factor.

Riboflavin

Widely found in nature, riboflavin is synthesised in the horse's intestine and is a factor in the metabolism of energy.

Deficiencies are associated with roughness of the coat, conjunctivitis and lacrimation.

Folic Acid

A component in the formation of red cells, folic acid is commonly added to equine feed supplements. It is also synthesised in the equine gut.

A vitamin of the B complex, closely associated with vitamin B12 in metabolism, deficiency can cause a form of anaemia. There is an increased need for folic acid in horses in training. Green forage legumes are a rich source. Supplementation can sometimes have beneficial effects.

Biotin

In carbon dioxide fixation, and in metabolism, biotin is intimately involved. The vitamin is universally available.

Like folic acid, biotin derives from the B vitamin complex. However, it is in an almost completely unavailable form in wheat, barley, milo (sorghum) grains and rice bran. Biotin in oats is only slightly more digestible; in maize, yeast and soya bean it is accessible, as it is also in grass and clover foliage.

Horses with hoof walls that tend to crumble may respond to biotin given over a period of 9–12 months in daily amounts of 5–10mg for ponies, 15mg for riding horses and 30mg for heavy horses. The strength and conformation of the hoof should also improve and 1–3mg daily is adequate thereafter.

Vitamin C (Ascorbic Acid)

The horse can synthesise vitamin C in the liver. It is important to the maintenance of healthy epithelium. Fresh fruits are a good source, as are greens including grass. Body requirements for vitamin C are normally met by synthesis from glucose and if there is a need for supplementation in horses it is only of use when given intravenously (5–10gm) as it is poorly absorbed from the gut.

Deficiencies are thought to cause a greater tendency to wound infection, epistaxis, strangles, viral pneumonia and performance problems in trotters.

Niacin

In glucose metabolism niacin is essential. Brewer's yeast is a good source, but it is also considered to be synthesised in the equine gut. In other species deficiencies of niacin have resulted in mouth ulceration and bad breath; dermatitis has also been a feature.

Vitamin B6 (pyridoxine)

Widely available in nature, vitamin B6 is active in protein metabolism. Deficiencies are unlikely under normal dietary conditions.

Pantothenic Acid

Although universally found, pantothenic acid is a nutritional essential active in all live tissues. While deficiences are rare, dermatitis, enteritis and diarrhoea are recorded symptoms in other species.

Choline

Universally available, choline is active in metabolism. As is the case with many vitamins, research relating to dietary requirements in the horse is sparse, but gut synthesis in horses makes it highly unlikely that deficiencies of choline will occur.

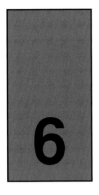

6 Defences Against Disease

The digestive system, not unlike the respiratory system, is an open portal for the entry of infectious organisms and other foreign, and noxious, material into the body.

Especially in grazing animals, the extent of contact with a whole range of bacteria, as well as internal parasites and other organisms found at ground level, is almost unlimited. It is therefore essential that such exposed body systems have protective mechanisms to offset the risk and ensure that life can continue.

Protective Mechanisms

With regard to the digestive tract, nature has developed a comprehensive defensive system, which, however effective, is not foolproof. Infections do occur, as every horse owner knows, and bacterial, viral and parasitic problems manage regularly to become clinical, especially in intensive conditions – the lesson to be learned from modern horse care and management.

Chemical Defences

Saliva contains the enzyme, lysozyme, which has the propensity to destroy organisms (mostly of a bacterial or viral nature). In the stomach, the sheer acidity of the medium is capable of destroying large numbers of organisms. However, there are other organisms which are not affected by acid conditions and are able to proliferate. Some, as we have seen, are beneficial; others are harmful.

The lining membrane of the stomach and bowel contains chemical substances, as well as antibodies, the purpose of which, again, is to defend the body against invasion.

There are also cellular defences of the blood system, brought to destroy foreign matter that escapes into the circulation. The complexity of the whole defensive system is thus significant. Some important aspects of this, unique to the bowel, are elaborated on in this chapter.

Mucus Coat Protection

A coating of mucus forms over the lining of the tract and so acts as a physical barrier to bacteria and their toxins and prevents many organisms from binding to surface cells.

The mucous membrane (right) *in the bowel and* (below) *detail of the finger-like villi which increase the surface area for digestion*

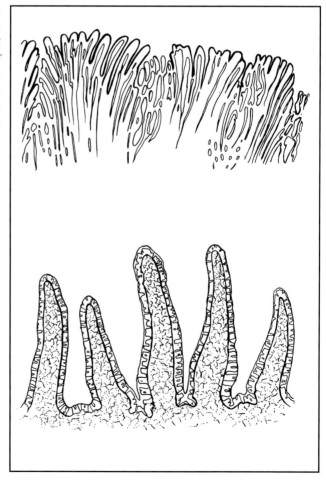

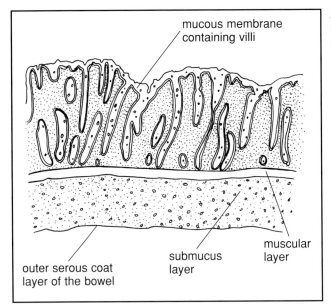

Diagram showing cellular layers of the bowel

mucous membrane containing villi

outer serous coat layer of the bowel

submucus layer

muscular layer

Mucus can occur as a thick, sticky gel, or as a viscous fluid, forming an unstirred layer. Some organisms, however, bind tightly to the mucus and are able to survive longer in this coated condition. Secretory immunoglobulins (antibodies) can also become incorporated into the mucus layer, adding to its protective capacity.

The lining of the stomach is itself protected from digestion (by acid and pepsin) by this layer of mucus. It lubricates the mucosa and also the luminal contents. Surface cells also secrete bicarbonate ions which neutralise any acid that penetrates the mucus layer.

In the normal course of events, surface epithelial cells are desquamated (shed) every two to four days and are able to spread rapidly over areas of denuded epithelium (resulting from chemical, infectious or mechanical insults).

Other Protections

Although the lining surface of the tract is exposed to a variety of foreign substances, access to the interior host tissues is limited. This is achieved by a barrier that includes the mucus layer, the surface cells, local antibodies, and chemical- and blood-borne cellular elements.

On the surface of the epithelial cells is a filamentous material that hinders passage of bacteria through their substance. Lymphoid tissue in the wall of the intestine is part of the same complex defensive system.

Intestinal plasma cells secrete antibodies, the influence of which may inhibit potential organisms at the portal of entry to the wall of the intestine. Similarly, produced antitoxin can neutralise toxins from bacteria before they enter the systemic circulation.

Peristalsis

The mechanism by which food is propelled through the gut, peristalsis, may, by the sheer turbulence it creates, act to dislodge organisms that are not tightly attached, or prevent others from becoming attached.

This benefit is augmented by desquamation of cells from the surface of the bowel when there is heavy bacterial growth, thereby inhibiting invasion into deeper layers.

Naturally Occurring Bacterial Protection

The lining of the stomach and bowel provides an ideal medium for the growth of micro-organisms. These latter are acquired within hours of birth from the immediate environment and from the dam of the newborn foal and become established as the normal flora of the gut. As many as 1,000 million bacteria per gram of food material are found in the caecum and colon; and as many as 400 different types of bacteria may exist harmoniously within the tract.

Foals, coming as they do from the sterile environment of the uterus, have a developing flora within 48 hours, consisting of organisms such as *E. coli*, streptococci and lactobacilli.

The type of organism in the established flora of the mature horse varies, but can be dictated by the nature of the diet, being loosely divided into lactic acid fermenters, non-fermenters and coliforms. Ensuing from this, a sudden change of diet may be met by a population of bacteria unable to digest it, leading to an acute digestive crisis, perhaps diarrhoea and death.

Organisms attach to lining cells by means of substances known as 'adhesins'. Colonisation of the tract by disease causing (pathogenic) organisms (for example, *Salmonella*) is greatly impeded by the indigenous flora and any prospective pathogen must be able to adhere to the bowel wall in order to compete. If they fail to do this, they are swept away in the intestinal fluids. Various other similar factors also protect the bowel from infectious bacteria, a significant example of which is the acidity of the stomach, or that caused by fatty acids in the colon.

Microbial by-products are a means by which the indigenous flora functions to maintain a constant population of organisms, existing in a symbiotic (mutually beneficial) relationship with the host. Some bacteria produce antibacterial factors called bacteriocins. Colicins, for example, produced by *E. coli*, can kill other members of the same species, thus protecting their ground. There is also produced a protective mechanism for the cell that produces it. Production of fatty acids as a by-product of anaerobic metabolism helps to create an environment toxic to some bacteria. Small intestine (enteric) bacteria thus become less numerous in the colon should it be colonised with anaerobes. The low (5–6) pH of the colon makes the environment hostile to organisms that thrive in the more alkaline small intestine and these will not readily colonise.

A lack of required nutrients can limit the ability of an organism to colonise the tract, be these beneficial or hostile to the host; and implicit in this, again, is the need for dietary consistency in order to avoid sudden digestive upsets. The indigenous flora may have to compete for an essential source with a potential pathogen. The result is disease should the pathogen take over.

One role of the bacterial flora of the newborn foal is to prime the gut for its future as an immunologic organ, protecting the animal from invasion by unwanted organisms. Exposure to bacteria causes proliferation of defensive lymphoid cells within the lining of the gut and these act at all future times to prevent unwanted colonisation.

It thus follows that the normal bacterial flora acts as a barrier to invasion by pathogenic bacteria. However, the use of antibacterial drugs can eliminate the resident flora and allow overgrowth of bacteria resistant to the drug.

Resistance to an antibiotic is commonly acquired and can be transferred between bacteria, and the drug may then become useless against a range of bacteria. Resistant bacteria may then become the predominant flora after prolonged therapy. The obligate anaerobes (which grow in the absence of oxygen) and other susceptible bacteria are often replaced by pathogenic organisms. This situation may be complicated by the development of yeast or fungal infections, which the normal flora usually keeps in check.

Responses to Parasites

The invasion of the gut by parasites is different because the type of organism encountered is not a single cell structure but a much bigger entity, often with biting mouth parts and a capacity to tear away sections of the bowel lining, perhaps then entering the circulation, or other body

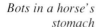

Bots in a horse's stomach

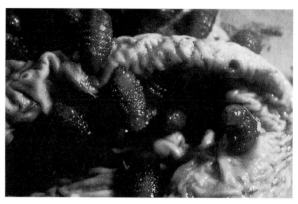

tissues, as part of its life-cycle. The influences of this type of disease, especially where heavy infestations may cause extensive damage to the bowel, are self-evident; although the problems created by pathogenic bacteria can be more immediately destructive to the host.

Parasites of the bowel affect digestion both by the direct damage they do to surface tissues and also by competing with the host for the benefit of ingested food material. They may also, because of physical bulk, limit available digestive space, aside from any effect they may have on digestive secretions. As an example of this, it is not unusual to see an animal's stomach distended with bot larvae in those horses slaughtered at the appropriate time of the year. Furthermore, extensive damage to surface tissues may inhibit the production of digestive enzymes.

The body's response to infestation is local inflammation, production of antibodies, and a gradual development of immunity as the animal is exposed. This reaction can often be acute and greatly add to the severity of disease and significantly contribute to the quantity of fluid (and protein) lost from the body.

A local anaphylactic reaction is responsible for the phenomenon of self-cure, which takes place after a high intake of infective larvae, over a period of time. Release of antigens from the worm are thought to trigger the response from the host.

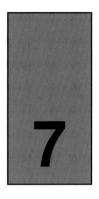

7 Signs of Disease

Disease of the digestive system is expressed in a number of ways. Locally inflamed areas may arise as a result of physical impediments to the digestive processes. A typical example would be hyper-acidity of the stomach, which might eventually lead to ulcer development. Equally, excessive gas production would lead to colic, or sudden changes in the bacterial flora might result in acute infection, perhaps expressed by sudden onset diarrhoea. The possible range of symptoms is, therefore, varied.

Clinical Signs

The first signs of digestive disease noted are likely to be pain (in colic), or diarrhoea, constipation, and the like. It is important to consider these in detail, though they follow in alphabetical form, rather than in order of importance.

Abdominal Pain

The horse has a number of ways of indicating abdominal pain, varying from the dull, depressed state seen with some forms of impaction to the acute, and often violent, response to twisted gut. In many situations, however, there is a tendency to recumbency, pawing the ground when standing, or continually getting up and down; sweating is associated with acute pain. An exception to this is the pain caused by peritonitis, which may cause the animal to stand rigidly without moving. It is usually not difficult to relate the source of pain to the abdomen, and the variability of signs and the intensity of reaction will lead the vet to decide the course of action to be taken. The need to control an animal's own violent reaction to pain is a priority as untold damage can be caused, which may be more serious than the original condition and may also mean the problem becomes incurable as a result.

Abdominal Swelling

Swelling of the abdomen often means there are excessive amounts of solid, fluid, or gas, in some part of the bowel. This may exist within an organ (for example, the stomach or caecum), or it may result from a growth, or from the presence of excessive quantities of fluid within the peritoneal cavity.

The most commonly seen swellings are associated with colic-type symptoms and may be caused by obstructions that prevent the normal flow of ingesta through the bowel. The production of excessive quantities of gas may exacerbate a less serious disturbance and cause pain that will only be alleviated when the gas has been passed, dispersed, or released.

Anorexia

A partial or total reduction of appetite may well be an indication of anorexia. The animal may continue to drink, or may drink to excess, but it may well also be that the anorexia is a symptom of diseases located in systems other than the digestive system.

Failure to eat, too, might be an indication of anxiety in an animal; for example, one that has recently changed ownership. This lack of appetite could also indicate an inability to eat.

Constipation

As a symptom of digestive disease in horses, constipation is not uncommon. In the uncomplicated state, it is an expression of indigestion.

The condition may vary from a barely noticed tendency to excessively hard and dry faeces, with no evident illness, to hard, mucus-coated, faecal pellets that may eventually require laxative, or stronger, drugs to move them. Constipation should not be confused with the situation when the bowel is obstructed and faecal material is sparse and hard, with a copious coating of mucus, but eventually stops completely when no material is passing the site of obstruction.

On a lesser scale, it has long been recognised that the retention of dirt, sand, soil, and the like) within the large bowel is an impediment to efficient digestion, especially in horses that have been stabled for long periods. In previous years, the idea of a weekly mash was an effort to relieve this. However, a condition marked by loss of physical condition, bad coat, perhaps impaired performance, was often treated to more drastic purgation. While it may be argued that such a scenario is an expression of inefficient bacterial digestion and some success is claimed with the use of probiotics, there are still animals suffering in this way that respond best to purging. Whether or not purging also leads to the establishment of a more balanced flora has yet to be explained, but is entirely possible. There may also be a significant influence on absorption, and electrolyte balance within the body.

Diarrhoea

Marked by an increased fluid content of faeces, diarrhoea is usually also associated with increased frequency of defaecation. There may also be abnormal colour and smell to the faeces.

Equine faeces normally becomes more fluid when grass is lush, or when horses are fed on laxative substances such as bran or sugar beet pulp. The difference between what are normal variations and what is clinical is not difficult to decide, however, especially as a horse with diarrhoea will have other symptoms – dehydration, depression, perhaps excessive water intake, and so on.

Dysphagia

When an animal has a clear interest in food but is unable to eat, or to swallow, dysphagia exists. Food may be taken into the mouth, but the animal is incapable of swallowing it. This could be caused by an obstruction, by injury, or by inflammation in the region of the larynx, by the presence of a foreign body in the oesophagus, or the animal may simply be unable to chew its food due to a painful tooth, or broken jaw. Food may be dropped from the mouth, unchewed, or there may be copious amounts of saliva returned from the nostrils, as is usual in choke.

Changes of Temperament

Horses with digestive diseases may suffer changes in temperament. This condition may vary from depression or dejection to violent responses to pain. Animals with acute colic are often in such pain they become violent. This violence is more often aimed at themselves rather than a handler, but

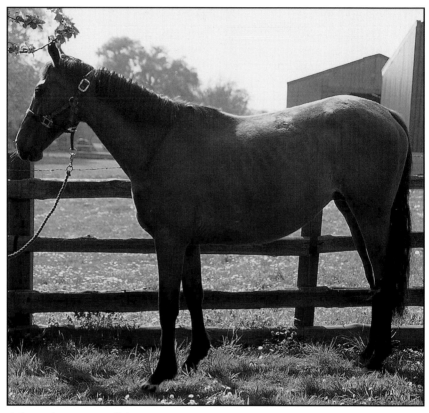

A horse in poor condition

the animal may have little regard for the safety of those who are trying to help. Head-pressing, incoordination and lethargy are frequent signs of liver disease, but many chronic bowel conditions can have similar effects, the symptoms being created by systemic and central reactions to an original problem.

Vomiting

Although vomiting is considered to be an unusual phenomenon in horses, that is not to suggest it does not happen. In fact, vomiting sometimes occurs as a feature of acute colic and it is suggested that this indicates increased pressure within the abdomen, or that vomiting may be a symptom of gastric distension, or rupture.

While gastric rupture would have serious implications for the future of the horse, not all vomiting indicates such a cause and the symptom may be relieved by the use of pain-killing or antispasmodic drugs, or perhaps, a combination of both. The decision will be made by the vet attending the animal, as will the judgement on what should be done next.

Weight Loss

In acute diarrhoea the onset of weight loss may occur very quickly, but it is as likely to be the consequence of chronic conditions (such as parasites) in the absence of diarrhoea. Weight loss may also result from conditions in organs other than the bowel – and for this reason, has to be taken into perspective along with other symptoms when a diagnosis is being made.

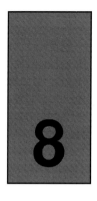

8 Diagnosis and Treatment

The diagnosis of digestive diseases involves a combination of clinical examination supported by specialist technology and, where necessary, laboratory tests. However, the first duty of the veterinary clinician is a complete physical examination of the animal, looking, to a certain extent, for symptoms an owner might well be able to help with – for example, the animal's temperature may have been taken and significant changes, in either direction, would be of concern.

History is very important: when were signs first noted, how long was the animal off food, showing pain, breathing heavily? The frequency of defaecation, and urination, might be important, as well as any evident changes in the colour, smell and consistency of either. The vet will also be interested in abnormal internal signs, like excessive gurgling sounds, evident swellings, heart and respiratory rates, and the colours of surface membranes. An internal examination, per rectum, may also be carried out, the scope of which is valuable, even if restricted by physical limitations, like the length of the arm relative to the animal's abdomen.

Treatment will usually be provided, or prescribed, on the basis of symptoms. However, treatment may only provide temporary relief from pain. It may be necessary to take samples for laboratory examination. Such samples will include blood, faeces, urine, abdominal fluid. Many clinical conditions are not diagnosed unless this help is to hand.

Diagnostic Techniques

Specialist equipment, using endoscopy, radiography, ultrasonography, and their like, are used, as well as procedures such as paracentesis, laparoscopy, biopsy, and blood analysis. However, the practicalities of equine medicine mean that clinical opinions are a priority and that treatment is routinely initiated before tests can be processed. A horse with colic needs immediate relief from pain, perhaps measures to counter dehydration, and also efforts to relieve the cause. The clinical examination must attempt to locate the source of the problem and treat it, as long as it lends itself to treatment. However, samples for testing may be taken at the same time, to help diagnosis, to gauge the influences on other body systems, and to decide what further treatment is required, including the need for surgery or otherwise.

Endoscopy

The development of the fibreoptic endoscope has seen a revolution in the diagnosis of respiratory, digestive and reproductive conditions, especially in human medicine. These costly instruments contain small glass fibres for transmitting light and image and may also have electronic imaging systems that allow a picture of remote tissues, (the stomach, for example) to be viewed live on a television screen.

An endoscope allows direct access to tissues which otherwise could not be inspected, and without a need for surgery. Tissue samples, or biopsies, can be taken from areas under examination, like the stomach and duodenum, and the instrument can be guided in different directions as well as having channels for air insufflation and suction. Samples of fluid may be taken from formerly inaccessible sites for microscopic examination and further laboratory tests.

In equine medicine, use of this equipment is influenced by the size and nature of the animal, as well as, of course, the demand for such services in what is a relatively small industry, where cost is an immediate consideration. The facility is routinely used in racing practice, but with limitations. Endoscopy is important in examination of the respiratory system, especially the structures of the pharynx and larynx, but, in diagnosis of diseases of the lower tract, it relies to an extent on laboratory back-up, and on the experience of the operator.

In the diagnosis and management of digestive tract diseases in human medicine, endoscopy has established new horizons; in horse medicine, however, practical limitations mean that the horizons are less comprehensive. The length and diameter of an endoscope decides the extent to which the digestive system can be examined. To inspect the oesophagus in an adult horse, an endoscope of 180cm in length is required; 110cm will reach the upper oesophagus only. To examine the tract of a foal, a

A horse being scoped. The vet passes the endoscope into the horse's lungs, enabling visual access to be made

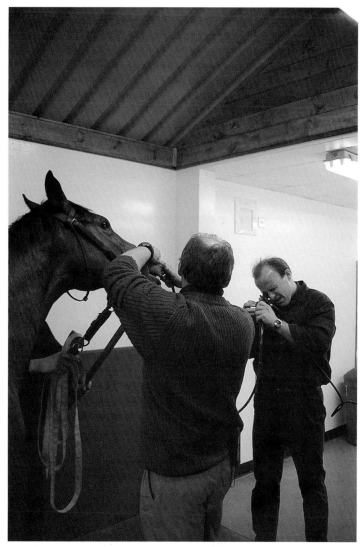

diameter of less than 10mm is needed. And 110cm will reach the stomach in a foal of one month old; some 150–180cm will reach the stomach of a weanling and 200cm is required to reach the stomach of an adult animal. A length of 200cm will reach a foal's duodenum up to six months of age; and between 275–300cm is required for duodenal examination of an adult horse.

Endoscopy, as in the human, requires, as far as possible, that the tract be empty, and that the endoscope be sufficiently flexible to make the various manoeuvres required. Examination of the rectum and distal small colon is also carried out and requires prior evacuation of faeces. Growths and other abnormalities may be detected and rectal biopsies may be taken. Sedation is generally used because of the nature of the intrusion and because of fears of penetrating the bowel.

Radiography

While radiography of the tract of foals is possible with normal equipment, stronger units are needed in looking at teeth, pharynx and the oesophagus of adults. Contrast media may also be used as well as varying views to achieve maximum differentiation of tissues. In young foals, meconium and faecal impactions, displacements, volvulus, stricture and congenital malformations can be detected through visceral distention and gas formations which are seen on X-ray.

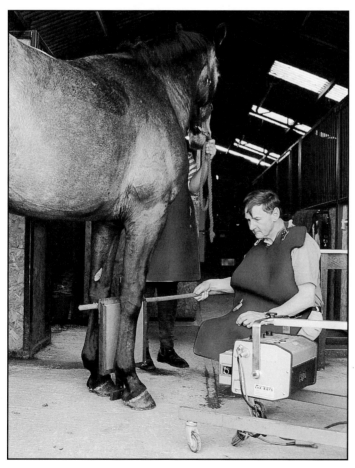

A horse being X-rayed

Peritonitis and abscess formation may also sometimes be seen. Barium is used for contrast of the oesophagus, stomach and proximal small intestine, also for the distal small colon and rectum. Enlarged oesophagus, stricture (narrowing) of the entry to the stomach, gastric ulceration, pyloric stricture, duodenal stricture and gall bladder conditions are all imaged in this way.

Ultrasonography

Diagnostic ultrasound is another miracle of modern medical technology. This type of scanning is used with considerable success in stud practice.

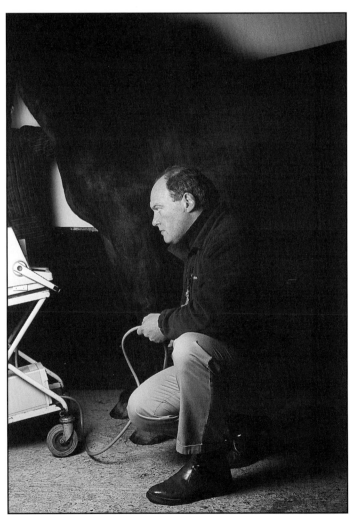

A horse being scanned

While its use is being developed in various other diagnostic spheres (heart disease and soft tissue injuries being the most significant), ultrasound has considerable limitations in dealing with abdominal disease. Depth of image is the problem and structures deeper than 20–25cm may be difficult to visualise. Interpretations are based on the manner in which transmitted sound waves are reflected by the tissues under examination. The technique is non-invasive and the animal has no sensation of what is going on. The sound waves are reflected back onto the working head and a picture is formed on a screen. This is interpreted by the vet, and it is possible to produce a photograph of the findings for record purposes.

The site for examination is clipped and a coupling gel used to enhance the contact between the operating head and the skin, and to eliminate air. Gas in the bowel stops the penetration of sound waves, but fluid does not. Peritoneal effusions may be diagnosed, as well as adhesions, abscesses, growths, dilatation of the duodenum, increased thickness of the bowel wall, dorsal displacement of the colon over the nephrosplenic ligament (cause of painful colic) and caecal impaction.

Paracentesis

By introducing a sterile needle through the lower abdominal wall, a sample of fluid may be obtained from the peritoneal cavity. In modern practice, this procedure, known as paracentesis, is frequently carried out by veterinary surgeons. It is of particular importance in non-responding colic.

The fluid sample, when examined under a microscope, reveals the presence of blood, cells, and bacteria, and will also show evidence of contamination with ingesta when the bowel has ruptured. Any of this information may be critical in deciding on the advisability of surgery, or other treatment for the various conditions that may exist.

It needs to be stressed that there are inherent risks (especially infection) in carrying out any procedure of this type. Vets are trained to anticipate these risks. There is no situation in which an unqualified person should ever attempt this type of intrusion on a horse.

Laparoscopy

The procedure known as laparoscopy involves entering the abdomen surgically, using microsurgery techniques, with instruments (like an endoscope) having a light source, insufflator and biopsy facility.

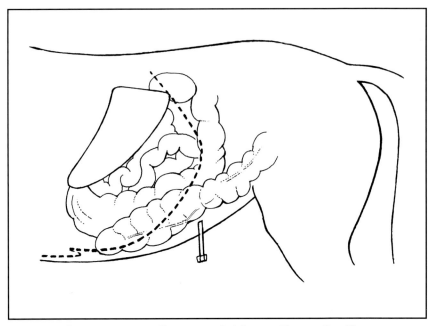

Diagram of paracentesis needle in ventral abdomen. The needle will not penetrate the bowel in most circumstances

Schematic diagram of laparoscopy – viewing the liver. The vet makes a minor incision, then passes the instrument into the horse's abdomen, enabling a visual examination for lesions, etc., to be carried out

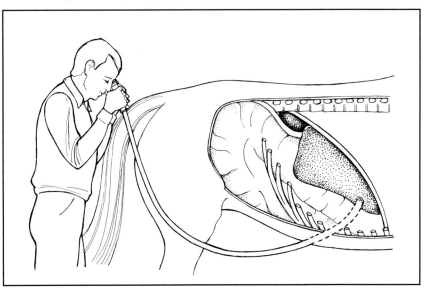

Laparoscopy is carried out after paracentesis, perhaps, and often to further investigate an abnormality detected already, as a result of ultrasound scanning, radiography, or manual examination per rectum. The nature of the intrusion, and the equipment used, will decide whether the procedure can be carried out using local anaesthesia and sedation, or if general anaesthesia is required. Very refined sedation techniques are available today, meaning far more examinations can be performed on the standing animal than was previously possible.

Biopsy

From the many tissues suspected of being diseased, biopsies can be taken and examined under a microscope at a laboratory. Thus, without great difficulty, biopsies of the stomach, duodenum, or of any abnormal tissue accessible to an endoscope, may be taken. Liver biopsies are taken under the guidance of diagnostic ultrasound. Many other tissues, including tumours and other growths, can be examined.

Rectal mucosal biopsy sections are taken with a uterine biopsy forceps. The information provided is limited because tissue changes in this area may not reflect the condition of the bowel at more critical anatomical sites. However, in chronic conditions, especially chronic diarrhoea, it is possible that cellular changes in the rectum may help in making a diagnosis and deciding on treatment.

Faecal Examination

The examination of faeces may provide information which can help in diagnosis. The consistency, colour, and state of digestion, are all important details, as is the presence of foreign material such as sand, or the like. Direct examination for parasites is carried out – bacteriology may well be critical in dealing with infectious conditions.

Loose, watery faeces with increased particle size suggests decreased colonic transit time. The presence in large numbers of white blood cells indicates an inflammatory process in the distal colon.

Occult blood may be detected where there are gastric ulcers or other haemorrhagic disorders of the tract. However, negative findings may occur even when there are large amounts of blood emanating from the proximal tract.

Faecal culture may produce organisms such as *Salmonella, E. coli*, and their like, and special tests may identify enterotoxic strains of organism. In addition, estimates can now be made of the normal gut flora, and the results of such tests often lead to better understanding of dietary influences and how errors might be corrected.

Rotavirus is detected in faecal samples using an ELISA test.

Digestion/Absorption Tests

Lactose is used to check the capability of the small intestine to absorb digestive material. A 20 per cent solution is used at a rate of 1gm/kg. If the bowel is working effectively, the serum glucose level should double in 60 minutes. Xylose is considered more specific and the test should be carried out after an 18–24 hour fast. Samples are taken every 30 minutes for four hours.

Blood Analysis

As an adjunct to the diagnosis of digestive tract diseases, blood analysis is used, and is very important, especially where there is dehydration, the risk of acidosis or alkalosis, as well as conditions such as protein depletion (from loss into the bowel, failure of absorption, etc.), anaemia, and interference with clotting.

Analysis of blood may be the most significant aid in deciding on the need for surgery in colic. It may also be critical in any post-operative treatment and in decisions made during recovery. In acute conditions, regular monitoring of packed cell volume (PCV), white blood cells (WBC), sodium, potassium, chloride, and tests for acidosis/alkalosis are made. PCV provides a close monitor on hydration, while WBC counts measure infection, allergy, etc. Red blood cell (RBC), PCV and haemoglobin (Hb) are all lowered in blood loss, but are raised where there is dehydration.

Many further tests exist that may help in providing a diagnosis, but it must be understood that all laboratory tests are merely a means to an end and are seldom capable of answering questions on their own. Clinical medicine is a combination of learning, experience and judgement, and a product of educated opinion coupled with information from those tests available in a particular situation. In the end, it is the human brain that must decide, depending on what has been learned from physical examination, and the results of tests and analysis. Even the most positive of results may be misleading if not properly interpreted. The finding of infectious organisms may still not mean the particular organism is causing disease. It is vital to keep these matters in mind. It is the clinician who must decide. That is what all the training is for.

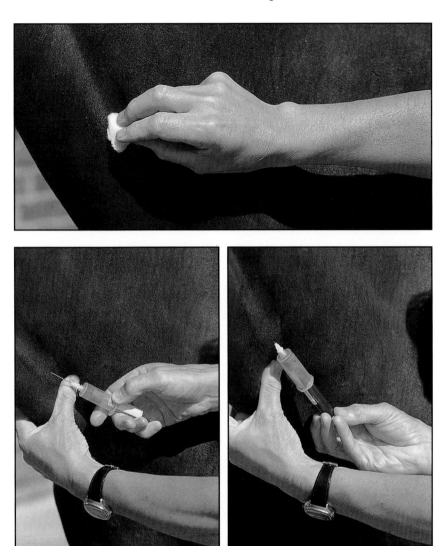

Taking a blood sample. The vet swabs the horse (top, left)*; inserts the empty syringe into the horse's neck* (above, left)*; and fills the collection tube* (above, right) *with blood*

Serum proteins provide a further guide to the presence of disease, or to the effects of disease on other body systems. There is a lowering of serum protein in some conditions of the bowel. There is also deficiency of immunoglobulin in foals that fail to achieve passive transfer from their dam in the first hours of life. These deficiencies can be detected on serum analysis. Plasma viscosity also provides a general guide to inflammatory disease; plasma fibrinogen acts as an indicator to tissue inflammation.

Further tests on serum can help to suggest more specific causes for disease.

Principles of Treatment

The first principles of treatment in diseases of the digestive system depend on whether the condition is infectious or non-infectious. Once the condition is diagnosed, there are various methods of treatment and some of these are discussed below.

Fluid Replacement

Saliva and intestinal fluid are naturally secreted in volume to assist the digestive processes as food passes through the gut. About 200 litres of fluid daily is made available in this way for an average 450kg horse. Most of this is reabsorbed through the caecum and colon, but the horse still requires somewhere between 12–36 litres of added fluid daily to balance natural losses, but this may be increased in fever.

Aldosterone (a hormone from the adrenal gland), produced as a result of fluid shifts that occur after feeding, promotes sodium and water absorption from the large colon. The affect of fluid movement from one compartment of the body to another like this is less marked when feeding occurs every few hours.

Fluid and electrolyte balance can be upset by lower intake or by intestinal disease – for example, obstruction, infarction (blockage of blood to or from a tissue) or enteritis. Obstruction prevents reabsorption and the earlier this occurs in the bowel (that is, the stomach and the small intestine), the greater the degree of dehydration.

Horses with infarction and strangulation suffer shock (caused by absorbed bacteria and endotoxin) and pooling of intestinal fluid. Endotoxin release can cause increased capillary permeability, resulting in protein and fluid leakage into tissues outside the vascular system and pooling of blood within the system itself. Overloading of lymphatics and

- Treatment of the cause in infectious conditions may require antibiotic use
- Probiotics may help to restore the natural gut flora
- Inflamed tissues are helped by controlling dietary intake and feeding intravenously
- Should the latter become necessary, fluid replacement therapy must be considered from the time symptoms develop
- Nutritive and digestible feeds are provided before normal rations are restored
- Appetite stimulants, and vitamins, minerals and amino acids may be administered
- Energy is provided through glucose or lipids in intravenously fed animals

Summary of treatment in infectious and inflammatory conditions

- Relief of pain, using pain-killing drugs, also sedation to prevent self-inflicted injury
- Gas accumulations are often eased by antispasmodic drugs
- Uncomplicated impactions are gently assisted by lubricant cathartics
- Complicated obstructions may require surgery; if so, fluid replacement therapy is critical
- Aftercare involves a gradual return to a normal diet

Summary of treatment in non-infectious conditions

impairment of capilliary function prevent the return of lost fluid to the bloodstream. If the dose of endotoxin is lethal, restoring blood volume is, inevitably, only a temporary relief.

Enteritis produces fluid, electrolyte and possibly protein loss from the bowel that may be acute or chronic. This occurs because of reduced absorption as well as increased secretion. Loss of fluid can be as much as 80 litres per day in conditions like *Salmonella* in adult horses, and this may cause acute electrolyte shifts.

Acid-base balance is controlled within the gut (see Chapter 3). Acid produced in the stomach is neutralised by bicarbonate contained in saliva and duodenal fluids; volatile fatty acids in the colon are dealt with in a similar manner. Enteritis, however, results in severe acidosis (of the blood) due to hypovolaemia (lowered volume of circulating fluid) caused by massive fluid loss.

The purpose of fluid therapy is, therefore, to restore circulating blood volume, to control acid-base balance, and to provide energy. Proprietary and commercial preparations are available to serve most of these needs, although there are clear distinctions between the ease of administration to a horse as opposed to, say, a human patient in hospital. Aside from the fact that compatible whole blood is not readily available in equine practice, the very physical problems of dealing with continuous intravenous administration are admirably dealt with; even where, on occasion, a groom has been left sitting on a recumbent horse all night, replacing drips as the need requires. Modern veterinary hospitals have the means and equipment to simplify this problem, although the vagaries of the animal have always to be taken into account.

Packed cell volume (PCV) and total protein (TP) are used as guides to hydration, but if blood loss or protein loss has occurred the information may be flawed. A horse in shock needs immediate balanced fluid in volume, especially if likely to endure surgery. Body water loss of 6 per cent (PCV 43–50, TP 7.0–8.2) or 10 per cent (PCV over 57, TP over 9.5) means slight to severe dehydration. On this basis, a horse with moderate dehydration might require 40 litres of replacement fluid to correct the immediate deficit, but, depending on the condition of the animal, some of this may be taken voluntarily, by mouth, with balanced electrolytes added. For example, the electrolytes most affected by bowel disease are sodium, potassium, chloride and calcium; magnesium and phosphorus to a lesser degree.

A normal horse requires a minimum of 36 kcal/kg per day of energy for maintenance only. A sick horse will require more than this, which may have to be given intravenously, using glucose or lipids (fats) as an energy source.

In all cases of water loss due to bowel disease there is a shift of sodium and corresponding water and sodium depletion is then likely to occur (especially marked in obstructive conditions of the small intestine).

Normal saline (0.9 per cent sodium chloride) is the most common fluid used in sodium replacement. If there is clinical dehydration without shrinking of the extracellular fluid (fluid that exists outside the body cells), due to loss of water without sodium, oral water or an oral glucose solution will suffice.

The provision of replacement fluids in diarrhoea is the most important aspect of treatment in non-bacteraemic horses. In foals, it is a critical adjunct to antibacterial therapy. These fluids may be given orally, where there is a reasonable expectation they will be absorbed. In any case of

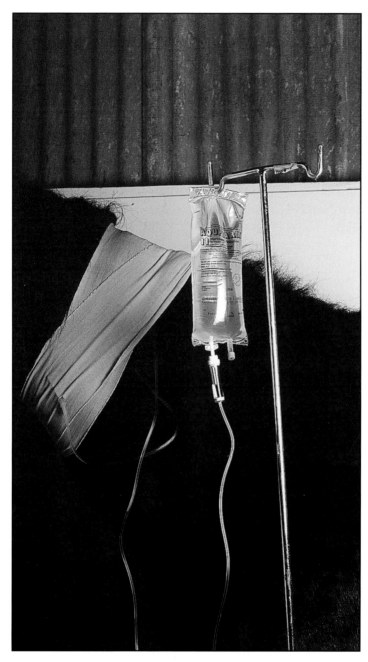

A horse on a drip. The needle is protected by the bandage and the length of tubing allows for a limited degree of movement

doubt, it is often best to begin therapy with intravenous fluids, which may be given continuously in very sick foals, and the vet will have to ensure the procedure for administration is both effective and sterile. The speed of administration will depend on the severity of the condition and the amount of fluid needing to be replaced.

Very often, depending on the results of blood tests, the vet will decide, from a range of balanced solutions, on which to use. The accent may be on sodium or potassium, and there may be a need to counter acidity or alkalinity of the blood. Through this fluid, there may be added B vitamins, glucose, amino acids, and so on.

Those sick animals able to drink voluntarily can be given balanced electrolyte solutions, administered by adding to water, in which case, drinking bowls are closed off in order to monitor intake. Electrolyte-enriched water can be provided orally by adding 30gm NaCl (sodium chloride), 12gm NaH2CO3 (sodium bicarbonate) and 5gm KCl (potassium chloride) per 4.8 litres of water.

Fluid can be given intravenously, orally, rectally or intraperitoneally. Balanced oral fluids are given in more chronic loss situations where absorption from the bowel is effective. If concentrated electrolytes are provided – for example, in paste form – then it is important that clean drinking water is readily available.

Large quantities of fluid are given intravenously using indwelling catheters. Water replacement is monitored clinically by mucous membrane colour and response to light finger pressure, also PCV and TP, skin torpor (gauged by pinching the skin of the neck), urine volume and body-weight.

In treating foals, drugs like loperamide (Imodium) may be of benefit in limiting fluid loss in diarrhoea, but are only an adjunct to fluid balance

Summary: other solutions which are used in replacement therapy

- Lactated ringers, which consists of calcium chloride, potassium chloride and sodium chloride in a balanced solution
- Acetated ringer's concentrate, consisting of sodium acetate, sodium chloride, calcium chloride and potassium chloride
- 5 per cent dextrose solution
- 4.2 per cent sodium bicarbonate solution
- Hartmann's solution, consisting of potassium chloride, sodium chloride, calcium chloride dihydrate and sodium lactate

and treatment of the underlying cause of the problem. These drugs inhibit secretion and increase water absorption (also electrolytes and glucose) from the intestine and are very useful in controlling symptoms.

Bowel Protectants

Bismuth, as a protectant, is used with limited success in diarrhoea, and may be given by stomach tube. Alternatively, activated charcoal is helpful in foals, but will need to be given in addition to antibiotics when a foal is bacteraemic.

Cathartics

Drugs that cause bowel evacuation are known as cathartics. The main indications for cathartics are: cleansing the bowel prior to radiography; helping to eliminate parasites after dosing; removing unabsorbed toxins from the gut; reduction of impaction; softening the contents in hernias or prolapses.

The drugs used can be grouped for our purposes under four convenient cathartic headings: irritant, saline, bulk, and lubricant.

Irritant cathartics

By stimulating smooth muscle in the wall of the bowel, irritant cathartics increase motility. Irritant cathartics include anthraquinones, cascara segrada, senna, aloin, and castor oil.

The vet will decide on the most suitable cathartic to use in any given situation, mindful of the limiting factors and risks. For example, irritant cathartics are not used in obstruction, enteritis or colitis, in late pregnancy or lactation.

Saline cathartics

Because both magnesium and sulphate ions are poorly absorbed, saline cathartics distend the bowel. This action causes movement of water into the bowel from extracellular sources. Peristalsis is increased by reflex action on the wall of the bowel. Saline cathartics include magnesium sulphate, sodium sulphate, magnesium oxide, and magnesium hydroxide.

Bulk cathartics

Administering bulk cathartics imbibes water into the bowel and thereby stimulates reflex peristalsis. Bran or linseed mashes can be helpful and often have magnesium sulphate (Epsom salts) added. Bulk cathartics include psyllium, methylcellulose and bran.

Lubricant cathartics

Both liquid paraffin and linseed oil are lubricant cathartics. Indeed, liquid paraffin may influence the absorption of fat soluble vitamins. However, it is commonly used, given by stomach tube, to foals with retained meconium, to assist with moving the obstruction from the proximal end. Adding an equal quantity of warm water makes the oil more easy to deliver through the tube.

Cathartics should only be given to horses with abdominal pain when it can be assured they will not further complicate the condition.

Antacids

The use of antacids in equine practice has increased along with the rising incidence of gastric and duodenal ulcers. Whether or not this ensues from the influence of diet, or rotavirus infection, the control of excessive acidity becomes important when it is likely to cause clinical disease.

While the whole range of human medicine antacids have been tried on horses, this is a developing area and new drugs are under research which will hopefully prove more effective in time. In the treatment of human bowel ulcers, antacids often only succeed in keeping symptoms at bay. Recent findings relating to the part played by *Campylobacter* and *Helicobacter* organisms have changed many attitudes in the approach to the treatment of this condition.

Drugs to Control Pain

The control of pain, by use of either central acting or peripheral acting analgesics, is a growing part of veterinary medicine. Some of these drugs are potentially habit-forming to human beings and for this reason are not available for use with horses, except through a vet. There is a whole range of drugs on this list, as well as drugs for sedation, and others for control of bowel motility (cisapride, used in human medicine, is proving useful).

Suffice it to say that pain control is possible, even if practitioners are often obliged to experiment by administering various depths of sedation to general anaesthesia. Suffering can be alleviated, and this is usually the first aim of the vet. However, there is some worry that using exceptionally strong analgesia may mask symptoms and in this way delay critical decisions regarding surgery until too late.

The effectiveness of acetylpromazine (ACP) as an antispasmodic has been largely undermined by exaggerated fears about its ability to cause prolapse of the penis in colts. This is one of the cheapest and most useful drugs available for use in spasmodic colic, especially, and it is in danger of being replaced by others that are not nearly as effective – and the use of which frequently allows the development of more serious problems, which may ultimately lead to the loss of an animal. This situation has evolved from the rising tide of litigation, and also from the opinions of so-called 'expert' witnesses in court.

The only indication for NSAID use in bowel disease is in endotoxaemia (or pain control in colic), but it is important to note these drugs may have adverse effects on an already inflamed gut.

Feeding

It should be recognised that irritated tissues will not be able to deal with food materials normally eaten. For example, grain intake should be limited in the aftermath of an inflamed gut, as should any indigestible food. However, good hay is frequently acceptable, especially as some roughage is needed to enhance the production of volatile fatty acids in the colon and to promote peristalsis. Foals may need to have milk withheld, by muzzling, and this is easily done with smaller foals. Access to the mare is controlled and the total consumption of milk reduced until there are signs of improvement. Plasma may also be administered to foals where there is any suspicion it is required – due to lack of protein as well as immunity. The plasma may be collected from the dam and given by intravenous injection as soon as the red cells have been separated.

A mixture of alfalfa or total diet pellets in water made into a gruel (5kg/per day) will provide a total maintenance nutrition for an adult horse.

Probiotics

The use of probiotics, or substances that foster the welfare of the normal gut flora, has been recognised since the turn of the century. For example, yoghurt, used extensively in human diets, contains the live organisms *Lactobacillus* and *Streptococcus*. The probiotic effects of yoghurt are well recognised and have proven efficacy in preventing and dealing with digestive infections, as well as increasing longevity in some investigated populations.

In horses, efforts to provide a normal gut flora in those animals suspected of having a sterile bowel were, in previous years, often carried out by means of strained faecal washes from normal horses, delivered by stomach tube. These efforts frequently proved effective.

Today, with a range of commercial probiotic preparations available, a greater rationale to therapeutic use has been established. Probiotics are prescribed where there is any risk to the existing normal flora – as might happen at times of dietary change, travel, excitement, and their like, or when antibiotics are being used.

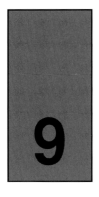

9 Non-infectious Diseases

For the sake of convenience, it is appropriate to separate diseases of the digestive system into those that are primarily non-infectious, those caused by bacteria and viruses, and those caused by parasites. In this chapter we concentrate on the non-infectious diseases. It is logical to begin with conditions affecting the horse's mouth.

The Teeth

Problems with teeth occur on a regular basis, beginning with hereditary and developmental conditions. The most common hereditary problem is parrot mouth (overshot jaw, where the upper incisor teeth sit in front of the lower incisors). The opposite effect (where the lower incisors rest in front of the upper) is called sow mouth. Parrot mouth is by far the more common of these two conditions.

Although a badly-deformed mouth can affect prehension, it is surprising how bad the condition may be in animals that never seem impaired by it – and never suffer from a lack of physical condition. However, the problem is hereditary and it is unwise to breed from horses affected in this way.

All sorts of abnormalities occur in the development of the teeth. Individual teeth may fail to develop, or grow at abnormal angles to the jaw. Generally, the problems that arise are not serious, although occasional surgery is required to remove teeth that are causing difficulties; for example, cutting into the cheeks.

When molar teeth are absent, there is a tendency for the opposing tooth to grow excessively. This may lead to painful injuries to the gum of the

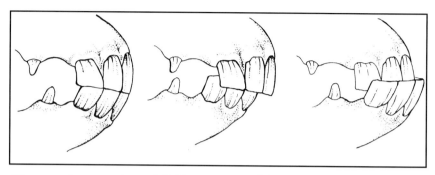

Diagram of: a normal mouth (left); *parrot mouth* (centre); *and sow mouth* (right)

opposing jaw and the only answer may be to remove the offending tooth, a task that will require general anaesthesia; or sometimes, the tooth may be cut back. On the other hand, where a tooth is missing, there is a tendency for food material to collect in the space created. This material will decay and develop a foul smell, sometimes resulting in infection of the local soft tissues, or causing neighbouring teeth to rot and, perhaps, have to be removed.

The most common ongoing problem with teeth is the matter of regular

Diagram of molar teeth, showing edges

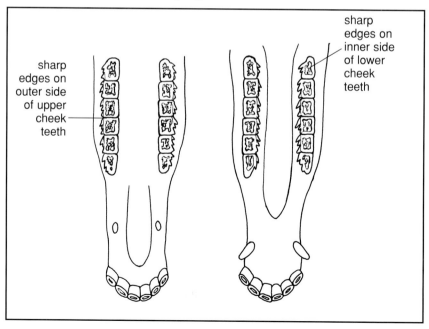

sharp edges on outer side of upper cheek teeth

sharp edges on inner side of lower cheek teeth

maintenance. The molar teeth, which are subjected to considerable grinding forces, have a tendency to wear in an uneven manner. The result is that sharp edges develop on the outer side of the upper cheek teeth and the inner side of the lower row. These edges may become so sharp that they cut into the cheeks and tongue and make the chewing of food a very painful process. The result is quidding of food from the mouth, or inappetance, and the problem can only be resolved by rasping away the sharp edges, following which the animal's chewing returns to normal.

Problems caused by the shedding of milk teeth do occur and it is sometimes necessary to remove a cap that becomes wedged between growing teeth.

Infections of the jaw, extending from the teeth, are not common, although they can occur. Frequently, these infections will require surgery to establish drainage and remove any rotten teeth, if they are causing the problem.

Dysphagia

The term 'dysphagia' means an inability to swallow, or a difficulty in doing so. It can also refer to problems with eating or chewing food. What is significant is that an affected animal may demonstrate a clear desire to eat, but is unable to do so – or is in such pain when it does that food is dropped from the mouth amid signs of clear discomfort.

Causes

Eating, an act that combines prehension, chewing and swallowing, depends on nervous control of the tongue and facial muscles together with sensory input from the mouth, lips and eyes. Damage, including paralysis, to any of these constituent parts may well be responsible for dysphagia, although damage to teeth or bones could also play a part.

Where facial paralysis occurs, the muscles of the lips, nostrils and cheeks are flaccid. The lip droops, food accumulates between the teeth and cheek, and may drop from the mouth. Horses affected on one side only may be able to eat enough to hold condition by using the other side. Damage to nerves takes a considerable time to correct itself, and there is little that can be done to reverse a process that is likely to take as long as six months before there is a return to normality. Inevitably, unless affected animals can be force fed, or manage to sustain themselves by other means, the outlook is very poor.

Lacerations of the tongue give rise to dysphagia, but do heal well. Infections of the tongue are not common in horses, though they may occur following wounds or the intrusion of foreign bodies. Dysphagia may be caused by poison (mouldy corn, lead, and so on), or by the effects of migrating parasites (for example, bot larvae invading the tongue). The problem sometimes happens after surgery. Fracture of the jaw would make jaw movement painful, as might gutteral pouch infection.

Strangles is marked in the early stages by pain in the throat area and inability to swallow. In tetanus, swallowing may be inhibited. Botulism is another infectious cause of dysphagia; rabies yet another. Yellow star thistle poisoning causes brain damage that results in paralysis of the tongue.

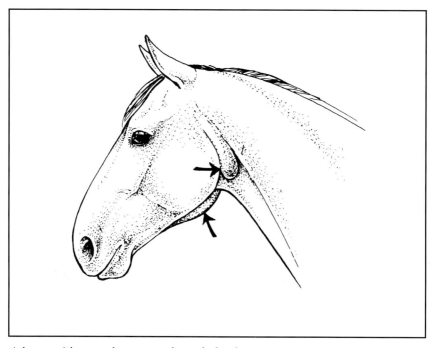

A horse with strangles, note enlarged glands

Dental disease may result in chewing problems. Tooth eruption and shedding of milk teeth can cause temporary soft tissue discomfort, also, as already said, sharp edges on the molar teeth can injure the cheeks and tongue, having a similar effect.

Local swelling of the mouth or pharynx may arise after stomach tube intrusions and use of a balling gun. Pieces of swallowed wood could also cause serious problems of dysphagia.

Clinical Signs

The difference between anorexia and dysphagia is the interest shown in food. An animal with anorexia has none, whereas a dysphagic animal is often hungry but unable to eat.

There are signs of varying degrees of discomfort, depending on the underlying cause. A horse developing strangles shows all the hallmarks of a sore throat, while one that has a piece of wood lodged in its mouth might be very distressed. There may or may not be a nasal discharge, and salivation is a frequent consequence of physical injury caused by foreign bodies.

Dysphagia of pharyngeal origin might lead to nasal reflux. Respiratory complications, too, might exist due to the entry of food into the trachea. Alternatively, material may collect in the pharynx and be coughed out through the mouth.

Horses exposed to yellow star thistle or Russian knapweed are unable to eat food or pass it to the pharynx but can swallow material placed there. Those suffering from this condition may want to eat and bury their heads in food or water and try to ingest it.

Diagnosis

In making a diagnosis the first step is to detect the underlying cause of the problem. Can the horse grasp food and move its mouth? Is the horse able to chew? Is there a cough? Are there signs of food coming back through the nostrils? There may be signs of expectorated food on the floor, walls, or in the drinking water.

Endoscopic and radiographic examinations of the pharynx, larynx, and of the gutteral pouches and oesophagus may be warranted.

Treatment

Inevitably, treatment will depend on the cause of the problem. Foreign bodies will need to be removed, often under general anaesthesia. Infections are treated locally or systemically, depending on their nature. Inability to swallow resulting from paralysis or poisoning will require, in animals that have a chance of survival, some form of artificial feeding until they are able to eat for themselves again. This could mean intravenous feeding, or repeated feeding through a stomach tube, as long as this option was practical.

No animal should be made to suffer unduly and the inevitable option is between futile efforts to sustain life and humane destruction, when this choice has to be made.

Oesophageal Obstruction and Choke

The purpose of the oesophagus is to facilitate the passage of food from the mouth to the stomach and prevent abnormal movement of any material back in the wrong direction.

The organ may be obstructed by objects, including growths, within its lumen, by stricture or narrowing, or by pressure resulting from external tissues or organs. However, the most common problem occurs when food boluses become lodged in the oesophagus during the process of eating.

Causes

Obstruction frequently arises when a greedy, or hungry, horse swallows something the size of a large potato without first crushing it with its teeth. It may also occur when there is competition for food and an inadequately lubricated bolus of hay fails to traverse the oesophagus. The same scenario may occur when grain or nuts are 'bolted'. Sugar-beet pulp is also a frequent cause. The most common finding in these cases is an enlargement of the oesophagus at the lower end of the jugular groove, just in front of the chest. The animal may be very agitated, with volumes of saliva being returned from the mouth and down the nostrils.

Blood in regurgitated saliva indicates tissue damage at the level of the obstruction and may indicate the presence of a foreign body. The oesophagus itself can be damaged by chemical or infectious agents and these possibilities need to be considered in diagnosis.

The whole oesophagus may fill and be clearly delineated. An acute onset suggests the animal has choked. Where the problem develops more slowly, other causes have to be considered. Weight loss might indicate a chronic nature to the condition.

Clinical Signs

If there is a choke, there will be severe salivation, evident pain, and the animal is disinclined to eat or swallow. Signs may be more subtle, for example, licking, agitation, colicky discomfort. Food material may return through the nostrils, mixed heavily with saliva and this may occur either immediately after eating of perhaps several hours later, depending to a degree on the nature and position of the obstruction. Mechanical obstructions may allow the passage of liquids but not solids, while if there are motility disorders (failure of peristalsis), food and water may be transported in the early stages of disease. Regurgitated fluid might equally come from the stomach or even the small intestine, if the blockage is sited there; in the latter case, evidence of bile would be significant.

In many cases there will be a bad smell from the animal's breath. It is often possible to palpate a swelling in choke and there is usually evident pain when it is touched. The animal is very uncomfortable, may wretch and continually shake its head and make swallowing efforts.

Diagnosis

It may be decided by the vet to pass a stomach tube, although the risk of perforation must always be considered; it is possible for a tube to penetrate or circumvent an obstruction without ever moving it, or to pass through a tear into surrounding tissues.

Radiography may be useful to identify the cause as the oesophagus is normally an inapparent organ on X-ray. The presence of air, fluid and food material would be significant and other foreign materials may be clearly defined. Barium sulphate may be needed as a contrast medium, given by mouth or through a stomach tube.

Endoscopy of the oesophagus is carried out under physical restraint or chemical sedation, for which purpose the fluid that precedes an obstruction may have to be removed by suction.

Diseases such as chronic organophosphate toxicity and grass sickness can result in a loss of motility in the oesophagus, thereby contributing to this problem.

Treatment

The immediate priority is removal of the obstruction. Where necessary, the relief of anxiety by using sedatives and pain-killing drugs may be required. Horses are very inclined to be distressed by pain and may react violently or suffer from shock. It is, therefore, very important to control symptoms and treat any significant dehydration. In many uncomplicated cases, the obstruction can be removed by using a stomach tube, but the dangers have to be constantly considered and it is not a course of action to be taken by anyone other than a vet. Liquid may be introduced through the tube (for example, water may help to push the obstruction forward, or liquid paraffin may lubricate it). This may alleviate the problem, though some, or all, of the liquid may be returned through the nose. The animal must not be allowed to feed. Visible impactions of the cervical oesophagus may be massaged; they do sometimes disperse. If there is a foreign body, general anaesthesia will be required in removal.

Afterwards, sloppy feeds are provided, though some animals return quickly to normal and show no further sign of the impediment.

Vomiting

In some species (like the dog and cat) vomiting is, perhaps, a protective mechanism and is preceded by nausea and retching. There is violent contraction of the diaphragm and abdominal muscles. In the horse, it is not considered to be a normal response, but is more likely to occur where there is distension and rupture of the stomach, a problem that may prove terminal in itself.

Ulcers of the Stomach and Duodenum

An ulcer is an erosion of the lining cells, leaving a raw circumscribed area, which may bleed. A perforated ulcer is one that runs the full depth of the bowel wall to the peritoneal cavity.

Ulceration is most common in foals, and is less frequently seen in adults, although there is considered to be a growing frequency in mature animals. The reason for this is not unconnected to modern feeding practices which are in danger of taking the horse further and further away from a natural diet. Ulceration may also be a sequel to serious infection with rotavirus.

In this chapter we will only consider the condition in the adult animal. Diseases of the foal are discussed later (see Chapter 12).

Causes

The lining of the stomach is protected by its coating of mucus as well as by the influence of bicarbonate in controlling acidity. While acid is essential to digestion, the potential danger it presents to delicate tissues lining the tract is not difficult to appreciate: excessive acid secretion is a recognised cause of ulcers, as is the enzyme pepsin. Delayed emptying of the stomach accompanied by prolonged contraction has also been blamed. It is possible that the time food material spends in the stomach is to some extent dictated by the nature of the food and the combinations of substances contained in the diet.

With the growing inclination for variety, there is a tendency for diets to become more complicated and for materials to be included that challenge the equine digestive tract (for example, when horses are first introduced to soya bean meal, their faeces may become soft, foul smelling and mucus coated, indicating inflammation of the tract). There is also a possibility when using pelleted feeds that individual constituents may vary in quality or origin, again leading to digestive upset. A lesson must be learnt from recent experiences with cattle. The equine digestive system is likely to work most efficiently, and with least disease, on diets that respect its basic needs.

Undigested, or improperly digested, food arriving in the duodenum, or excessively acid digesta, will result in inflammation of the lining, possibly leading to ulcers in that organ.

The greatest incidence of ulcers is found in horses in training, where diets may be complex and are, sometimes, fed to excess. The diet, using premixed or pelleted rations, may vary in quality, protein, or, indeed, in substances that make up the feed. While compounders usually insist on the consistency of their product, this is not always assured. And, for many other reasons (for example, the idiosyncracies of the feeder) horses may suffer sudden abrupt changes of diet and find their digestive systems unable to cope.

Inevitably, the greatest danger with changing food materials is to the bacterial flora of the tract. However, should food mixes interfere with the functioning of digestive enzymes, as is often suggested in human digestive diseases, the pathological effect could be accentuated in the stomach and small intestine. While there is no reason to believe the cause of ulceration in the horse has the same basis, the incidence is increasing, as are ever more complicated feeds that would never be encountered in nature.

Additionally, the common use of NSAID drugs is widely considered to be a cause of ulceration in animals on prolonged treatment regimes.

Clinical Signs

In adult horses there may be no apparent symptoms, and the condition may only be diagnosed post-mortem. However, there can be terminal, acute colic, with, perhaps, perforation of the gut. Alternatively, the horse may be in poor condition, constantly grinding its teeth, and generally showing signs of low-grade discomfort.

Diagnosis

Endoscopy is the best means of diagnosis and may be warranted where symptoms suggest the existence of ulcers and perhaps where faecal examination reveals the presence of occult blood.

Before endoscopy, so as to ensure an empty stomach, adult horses should not have been fed for ten hours. The stomach is insufflated with air to make the surfaces visible. A 275–300cm endoscope is needed for adults; and barium sulphate may be required as a contrast medium when radiographs are taken.

Treatment

The prime aim is to reduce or neutralise acid secretion. However, the pathology of the condition has to be taken into account as well as the cause; treating the symptoms is a short-term solution if the underlying cause has not been eliminated.

In other words, if the diet is causing the problem, immediate changes must be made. Remembering the animal is herbivorous, a diet of good grass and water might ease symptoms quickly, and provide adequate sustenance. Alternatively, good hay or silage might be suitable, perhaps with a little added oats if necessary. The quality of these materials is of great importance and any food likely to increase acidity or delay clearance times should be avoided. A stomach that is returned to an efficient working state is more likely to repair than one that has difficulty dealing with the food introduced to it.

The use of drugs to reduce gastric acid production is one that will have to be decided by an examining vet. While such drugs are in constant use in human medical practice, the indications for use in horses are not nearly as clear-cut, and effective drugs are still in the process of development.

Other Conditions of the Stomach

Gastric dilatation may occur from over-eating (for example, when a horse gains access to a feed store). Excessive water intake is also suggested as a cause. Dilatation may also occur as a consequence of blockage at the pylorus or in the small intestine.

Gastric impaction occurs if the stomach loses its ability to contract. This might occur with feeds that tend to swell after ingestion, or may result from improper mastication.

Gastric rupture follows either of the above and is sometimes marked by reflux at the nostrils.

Clinical Signs

Acute pain is common when the stomach is distended, although this may be followed by depression and shock, if it has ruptured. Peritonitis would be a natural sequel, although the condition could prove fatal, from shock, at an earlier stage.

If gastric contents are fluid, wretching may occur, and food may be vomited, coming out through the nares rather than the mouth.

When the stomach is dilated, horses have been known to assume a dog-sitting position to ease the pain.

In small intestinal blockage, there may be pooling of material in the stomach with eventual rupture. Pain is severe and continuous, pulse weak and thready, no peristalsis, no defaecation. Large amounts of fluid may be expelled on passage of a stomach tube.

Treatment

Rupture of the stomach is, obviously, extremely serious. While pain-killing and sedative drugs are essential to control the animal's reaction, patience must ensure that the situation is not compounded by adding bulk (through a stomach tube). If the stomach is overloaded from excessive eating, aside from treating the effects of dehydration and acidosis small amounts of mineral oil might soften the mass and help to move it on. However, this kind of interference carries a high level of risk and must only be attempted when the pros and cons have been evaluated. Where there is gas in the stomach, it may be relieved by the stomach tube and, in some cases, regular such relief is indicated. Rupture of the stomach would be detected on paracentesis, indicating a need for surgery, though chances of success would be limited, and some horses would be better saved from the misery involved in this procedure.

Malabsorption

When there are pathological changes in the lining of the horse's bowel, malabsorption occurs. This is especially so at sites like the small intestine, where digestion is active and selective, and where important minerals, for example, are absorbed through the wall. Taking calcium, for instance, this mineral is not absorbed significantly later in the bowel and it may be lost to the body if not taken in where intended. A similar problem may also arise if substances (vitamin D, for example) are absent, or if there is an excessive proportion of phosphorus in the diet.

Malabsorption might result, too, from tissue damage due to worm infestation, as, indeed, from any other form of inflammation to the lining of the intestine. Rotavirus infection is seen as a possible cause.

Treatment first involves detecting the consequence (for example, a deficiency), which may be corrected by supplementation, or by parenteral injection. It is vital to provide food materials in easily digestible forms, to eliminate factors from the diet which might prevent absorption of specific substances (again, for example, excessive phosphorus preventing absorption of calcium).

Finally, the health of the natural gut flora is also of prime importance, especially as bowel organisms may produce enzymes (for example, phytase to break down phytates and so release phosphorus for absorption).

Colic

The expression used to describe acute abdominal pain, colic is one of the most common causes of emergency attendance to horses. The source of the pain may be any part of the abdominal contents, in either the bowel or other organs. In diagnosing the source the vet will carry out a full clinical examination including, where feasible, an internal examination per rectum. However, it must be appreciated, in carrying out rectal examinations, that the vet is limited by physical parameters (a great part of the abdomen is out of reach of the human arm); also, it may be very difficult to examine any animal that is fighting pain.

Laboratory testing of blood and abdominal fluid may also be required.

Causes

The causes of colic are many but are best approached on a formal basis, appreciating that animal diseases do not always fall into easy patterns.

It is often the case that an animal suffering from colic changed pastures in the previous twenty-four hours, or there was recent rain, severe frost, or the animal was grazing lush, wet pasture. Spasmodic colic is common after rain in horses on lush grass, and may result from increased gut motility. Animals that eat frosted grass often show evidence of abdominal pain.

Many causes of colic are diet related, resulting, perhaps, from changes made too quickly, or by providing food materials that are not easily digested. In the autumn, when horses change from summer to indoor training regimes, the incidence of colic increases. This may be associated with dietary change and, especially, introduction to poor quality hay.

Diagnosis

A diagnosis of colic is easily made, based on the symptoms of abdominal pain and the distress it causes. However, in trying to localise the precise origin of the problem, it is vital, first, to provide the vet with a detailed history of events. Matters such as change of diet are critical, as well as current management procedures (type of feed, when last fed), recent wormings, and if there is a recurrent history of colic. It is important to know when the horse last passed droppings, their colour, frequency and consistency. When did it last pass urine? How long have symptoms been evident?

Low-level pain may signify the start of the problem, although acute pain is more typical and this may develop gradually from less severe symptoms. The horse may then paw the ground and thrash about, the degree of pain suggesting a more serious problem than actually exists. However, delays in relieving symptoms risk allowing an animal to injure itself, or to exacerbate the internal situation by throwing itself on the ground and rolling, probably sweating. Profuse sweating is never a good sign, although it only reflects the level of pain and different horses vary in their ability to cope with that. Continuous high-level pain, not responding to pain-killing drugs, usually indicates a serious situation (a twist is an example) and it is the level and persistence of pain that often provides the most significant evidence of the severity of the colic.

Heart rate and pulse strength are both vital indicators in diagnosis. Where the pain is acute but heart beats per minute do not increase, it is unlikely that any irreparable damage has been done and the condition may well respond to treatment. Where the heart rate increases to more than 52/min, the prognosis becomes more guarded; cases with a weak pulse are deemed poor risk for surgery and heart rates above 100/min are considered terminal.

Discoloration of mucous membranes usually indicates systemic complications. Abnormal abdominal sounds may be evident and swellings may be noticed, perhaps due to gas accumulation – but these also often respond well to treatment. An increased respiratory rate might mean systemic changes, though it may only be a reaction to pain.

If there are no abdominal sounds it is possible that the bowel has lost its motility. This is significant, because a paralysed gut is not capable of moving ingesta onwards; it may also lead quickly to the production and absorption of toxins. A decision will have to be made as to whether the problem is caused by a blockage and whether or not this can be relieved without surgery. The degree of pain, and signs of toxicity, will be critical in making this decision.

It is also important to know if a mare suffering from colic is in foal, a factor that will influence the choice of drugs that can be used. It might also mean the pain was emanating from the uterus.

On rectal examination, the vet may find the rectum empty if there is a blockage, and the glove may collect mucus or blood if the condition is of some duration. The tone and condition of contents in the terminal colon may indicate if there is constipation, accumulated liquid, or impaction. On the right hand side of the abdomen, the caecum may be distended and areas of gas may be detectable in the large bowel. The animal's reaction to manipulation may suggest where the most acute pain is located.

By means of paracentesis, fluid is drawn from the ventral abdomen through a needle. The normal fluid is clear, straw-coloured and does not clot. It becomes turbid in infection, may be blood-stained, or may be dark-stained, with a foetid odour, where the bowel has ruptured. If there is an interference with blood supply, as might happen in a twist or an aneurysm, the fluid protein level will be increased, but this would have to be decided by tests.

Impaction

While obstruction of the bowel may occur as a result of ingesting foreign matter, such as a plastic bag, this is seldom the case in horses. Instead, impactions are the result of local conditions within the bowel, possibly caused by simple changes to the diet. They may also result from narrowing (stricture) of the gut, a loss of motility, a growth, abscess or twist. Impaction may also result from inadequate dietary fibre.

The obstruction may be partial, allowing some passage of digesta through the area, or it may be complete, preventing any material to pass the point. A simple obstruction does not involve local blood supply, but leads to painful accumulation of food material, fluid and electrolytes, which could lead to shock, starvation and death if untreated.

Impactions of the caecum and colon occur with dietary change, poor

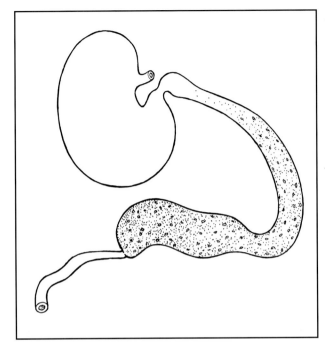

A schematic drawing of an impaction of the small intestine. The bowel beyond the blockage will gradually empty; that proximal to it will become enlarged as more food material arrives

hay, water deprivation, and teeth problems; sand is also a known cause. The diagnosis is made by rectal examination, when the distended organ is easy to palpate. Caecal dilation is a common cause of colic, but distension of the organ with liquid or gas may respond simply to treatment with sedatives or antispasmodics. The degree of pain in large bowel impaction is not acute and symptoms develop over a period of time. The horse will show varying levels of discomfort and may paw the ground and turn repeatedly to look at its flank. It may also be stiff and reluctant to move. In most cases, pain is easy to control and the impaction can gradually be moved by dosing with mineral oil by stomach tube, as long as the bowel is patent. But the untreated horse will be very uncomfortable until the condition is relieved, and symptoms usually do not abate without help.

Impactions of the stomach and small intestine are associated with much more pain and more likely to lead to rupture of the intestine, because of the size and nature of these organs. A great deal of harm can be done if there is any delay in making the diagnosis and initiating treatment.

Spasmodic colic
Probably the most common type of colic encountered, spasmodic colic results from gas-filled segments of bowel. These segments cause acute

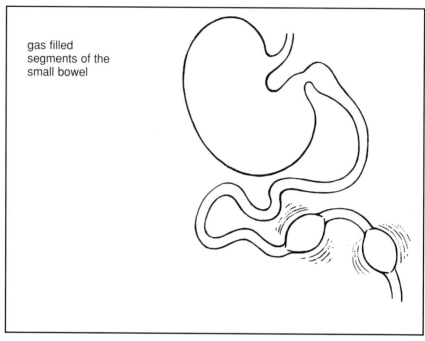

gas filled
segments of the
small bowel

*Schematic diagram of spasmodic colic. Excessive gas production may cause
local ballooning with acute pain*

pain, especially when touched during rectal examination. At times, however, the degree of pain the horse experiences can be so great that it
becomes impossible to distinguish spasmodic colic from twisted bowel.
Only response to treatment suggests the probable cause; and, of course,
there is nothing to say that a twist might not develop from a spasmodic
colic that has been untreated, possibly as a result of rolling.

Torsion, or twist

Twisted gut is, unhappily, a relatively common problem and frequently
can only be relieved by surgery. It is responsible for more deaths than any
other form of colic. It causes horrifying distress to affected animals,
responds poorly to pain-killing drugs, and is largely untreatable by medical means. Strangulation (the consequence of the intitial twist, perhaps)
involves compromise of the blood supply and may be confused with conditions that are primarily caused by blockage of blood vessels – such as
an aneurysm. Death results from fluid and electrolyte loss and shock
associated with absorption of toxins into the blood system.

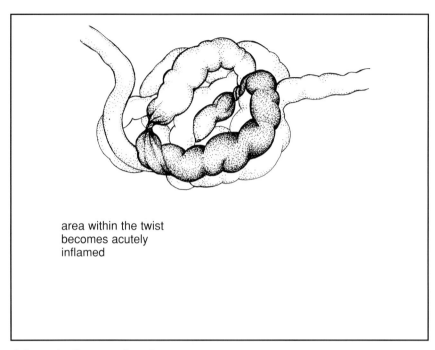

area within the twist
becomes acutely
inflamed

Schematic diagram of torsion

The first suggestion of twist comes with the poor response to analgesic drugs, an increased heart rate and injected membranes. The horse is in violent pain and may be too distressed to allow an internal examination to be performed with safety. It is likely to sweat profusely and may tend to collapse.

The general condition will include volvulus (twisting of the intestine), intussusception (telescoping of the intestine), rotation of intestine about its mesentery, and slipping of a section of intestine through a slit in the mesentery. All of these conditions result in interference with blood supply and inevitable obstruction, producing a situation that is irreversible except by, perhaps, completely removing the damaged section of bowel and creating a union between healthy tissues. Untreated, the animal will have no chance.

Worm-derived infarctions
In recent years, worm-derived infarctions have become less common, due to the advent of drugs of the type of ivermectin that kill strongyle larvae,

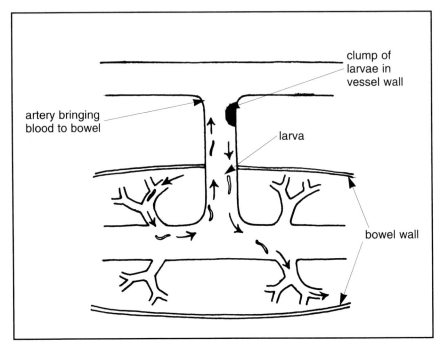

When a clump of larvae is freed from the wall of an artery it runs with the flow until eventually blocking a smaller vessel, thus causing an infarct by depriving the supplied area of blood

even when present in aneurysms within the blood vessels. The effect of emboli (clusters of larvae loose in the bloodstream) blocking vessels supplying the bowel is not necessarily very different from that of a twisted bowel. There is necrosis, meaning irreparable damage to the tissue deprived of blood. Depending on the size of the affected area, death is inevitable unless the animal can be saved through surgery.

The symptoms are very similar to those for twisted gut, with violent pain, increased heart rate, injected membranes. There is little or no response to drugs and animals sink quickly from shock and the effects of endotoxaemia.

Peritonitis and inflammation of the bowel

The cause of acute abdominal pain, peritonitis usually is associated with a temperature. The condition generally arises by extension from the gut, but could follow a puncture wound of the abdomen or even if infection is introduced by wandering parasite larvae. Diagnosis is made on the basis of the abdominal pain – which is generalised and causes the animal to stand rigidly and very tucked up – and the high temperature.

The condition may be confirmed by culturing abdominal fluid.

Inflammation of the bowel could result from poisoning with irritant substances (such as mustard seed) and the degree of pain this causes can be as acute as in severe colic. Dehydration, shock and toxaemia are natural consequences.

Treatment

It is not uncommon for vets to pass a stomach tube on animals with colic. However, this is not an automatic procedure and has to be based on good judgement. Frequently, the cause of the condition can be ascertained by external physical (and rectal) examination. Quick treatment may prevent the development of more severe symptoms.

One of the most serious consequences of acute colic is that affected animals may well injure themselves by violent behaviour. The result of this may, on occasion, be more significant than the colic itself. It is for this reason that colicky horses are kept on their feet and moving, and also prevented from throwing themselves on the ground or against hard objects.

Once the diagnosis is made, impactions are treated by controlling the pain and attempting to penetrate the impacted mass with lubricating substances such as liquid paraffin. If an animal is treated quickly, and the situation is not allowed to deteriorate, many will respond without complication. However, the addition of large volumes of fluid to an already distended gut can cause rupture and prove terminal, so that great caution needs to be exercised. Once the flow of ingesta is re-established, the health of the gut is restored by sensible feeding and by ensuring the bacterial flora is returned to normal.

Spasmodic colic is treated with the use of antispasmodic drugs and analgesics and usually responds quickly as long as the condition is uncomplicated. Acetylpromazine (ACP) is very useful in relieving spasm (but not recommended in colts or stallions) and its influence is quickly seen; it may be used in conjunction with an analgesic. Pain is lessened, and there is often a tendency for the animal to soon pass substantial quantities of gas per rectum and then begin to show an interest in food. Feeding good hay in small quantities is not harmful as the pain recedes, especially where the heart rate is normal and there are no other external signs of abnormality (such as unaccounted swellings). Laxatives are not necessary and use of a stomach tube is contra-indicated in this condition, except if fluid replacement is necessary for horses that have suffered excessively and, perhaps, are dehydrated.

Medical treatment of acute catastrophies like twisted gut are generally only of use in sustaining an animal until surgery can be performed. This will include the use of potent pain-killers, antitoxic drugs and the administration of intravenous fluids to counter the effects of shock, acidosis, alkalosis and dehydration.

Inflammation of the bowel is treated by removing the cause, promoting healing of the damaged tissues (which may be achieved by control of the diet), and restoration of the normal gut flora. The use of antibiotics will be decided by the vet, but is not an essential aspect of treatment today. In peritonitis, however, antibiotics are usually essential, and these are best based on sensitivity tests, especially in resistant cases.

If the stomach is dilated, passage of a stomach tube may relieve the immediate problem, but the procedure might need to be repeated, and pain must be controlled until the immediate crisis is over. Also, using a very stiff stomach tube could perforate tissues, especially if force is used as it goes down.

Surgery is indicated when there is severe pain that cannot be controlled, discoloration of abdominal fluid with, perhaps, blood, and, where there are indications of displacement, or twist, on rectal examination. However, in making a decision to operate, the future quality of life for the animal must be considered as well as the economics, and the likely chance of success. It has to be understood that the proportion of successful operations is not high, and many failures to save animals are due to delay before the decision is made. There are many other factors also to blame.

The vet has available a range of sedative, pain-killing and other drugs to treat the symptoms of colic. However, control of pain is only a first step and not a cure in itself. Flunixin meglumine is the most effective non-steroidal anti-inflammatory (NSAID) analgesic for control of visceral pain in horses, and its effect lasts for from 1–24 hours depending on the cause and severity of the pain. It helps reduce the effects of endotoxin absorbed from the bowel, but has toxic side effects similar to butazolidin, and is mainly criticised for its ability to mask symptoms of severe colic.

Fluid therapy is important for animals suffering prolonged colic and shock, and especially important if surgery is anticipated. Whether or not fluid therapy can be given orally or intravenously is a decision that will be made by the vet depending on factors relating to the individual case.

Magnesium sulphate is sometimes used as an alternative to liquid paraffin in mild impactions, given by stomach tube in about 4 litres of water. Psyllium hydrophilic mucilloid is a bulk-forming laxative that is effective and safe for horses. Dioctyl sodium sulfosuccinate is also used and is good in penetrating impactions.

- Impaction and other obstructions
- Spasm of sections of the bowel (spasmodic colic), usually due to local accumulation of gas
- Torsion, or twist, of part of the bowel
- Worm-derived infarctions (interfering with circulation)
- Inflammation of the bowel and peritonitis

Summary: the causes of colic

Paralytic Ileus

In paralytic ileus, the stomach, small intestine and colon are atonic and dilated. The problem arises following abdominal surgery, some disease processes involving the nervous system, and with the use of some drugs. It can also be a feature of peritonitis. Signs are of abdominal distension, reduced intestinal sounds, vomiting or reflux and dehydration. Ileus is described as a functional obstruction of the bowel and may be associated with inflammation of the small intestine or colon. It is clinically indistinguishable from mechanical obstruction requiring surgery. Bowel motility may be restored with infusions of calcium, magnesium, potassium, where these are shown to be deficient in plasma. Cisapride, a drug used in human medicine, has been found to be useful in countering this condition.

NSAID Toxicity

Diarrhoea is a common consequence of phenylbutazone toxicity. Doses of 8mg/kg per day for more than 4 days and 4mg/kg/day for more than 50 days have been associated with toxicity. Doses of more than 15mg/kg are uniformly fatal. Flunixin has been suspected of causing toxic effects at high doses.

There is weight loss, anorexia, depression, colic and varying degrees of diarrhoea. The condition can be compounded by using more NSAIDs in therapy. Mucous membranes are injected and there may be ulcers on the lips, cheeks or tongue. Abdominal distension may occur and is associated with ileus; there may be ventral oedema. Ulcers contribute to the anorexia and may be present in the stomach or duodenum as well, resulting in teeth grinding and bloodstained loose faeces. Ulcers of the colon cause more acute abdominal pain and fluid diarrhoea. Perforation may lead to peritonitis. In severe cases, toxaemia is profound and it may be impossible to control pain. Blood and protein are lost from the gut.

Diagnosis is based on the history of drug exposure combined with the symptoms.

Fluid therapy is important and also treatment for ulcers by control of diet and drugs to counter acidity in the stomach and small intestine.

Mild cases recover without complication, but more severe cases are often fatal.

Heavy Metals and Other Poisons

Heavy metals, such as arsenic and lead, may cause enteritis and diarrhoea, as might insecticides of the organophosphorus or carbamate classes. Arsenic can cause weakness, depression, diarrhoea, tenesmus and muscle tremors. Ensuing enteritis will cause bleeding and the course of the disease is short.

Organophosphate and carbamate poisoning will result in salivation, contraction of the pupil, lacrimation, diarrhoea, urination and pallor. Often the toxicity is mild and the diarrhoea transient.

Blister Beetle Poisoning

The blister beetle (*Epicauta spp.*) has been a cause of poisoning in horses in the United States. It is a leaf and flower feeder that swarms in hayfields. The source of poisoning is usually alfalfa hay. The active principle, cantharidin, which will blister the skin, is contained in the lymph and genitalia of adult beetles, which feed on alfalfa in mid- to late-summer. If the beetles are trapped or crushed in the hay-making process, the poison is released onto the hay which may remain toxic for years. Low levels of contamination are enough to cause colic. The minimum lethal dose is less than 1mg/kg hay.

Symptoms vary from anorexia and depression to shock and death. The poison may blister the tongue and create profuse salivation and severe abdominal pain. The horse may strain to pass urine, which may contain blood, faeces may be bloodstained, and diaphragmatic flutter is sometimes heard. There may be fever, increased heart and breathing rates and sudden death.

Diagnosis is based on chemical analysis of gut contents or urine. For a definitive diagnosis the toxin must be isolated and identified. On post-mortem examination there is ulceration and erosion of tissues in the oesophagus, stomach and intestine, also the bladder and the ventricle of the heart.

Affected horses are treated for shock and fluid loss. Protection of the bowel might be assisted by the use of aluminium hydroxide or activated charcoal. Liquid paraffin is sometimes used to clear the toxin from the gut. Mortality can be as a high as 60 per cent but most horses that survive 72 hours are safe.

Grass Sickness

A disease of unknown cause, grass sickness does appear to be confined to particular areas, although this may be a developmental aspect in the path of the disease. In recent times, cases have been reported on an ever-widening basis.

Causes

It is suggested that grass sickness is caused by an ingested poison that damages parts of the nervous system, resulting in partial paralysis of the intestine. The condition is, as the name suggests, most commonly seen in grazing horses, although young horses being moved from stables to grass are known to be at risk. The precise nature and identity of the causative agent is unknown.

Clinical Signs

Acute and chronic types of the disease are recognised. Acute cases may be found dead or in an incurable condition, lasting no more than one to two days. Severe colic is common, possibly a ruptured stomach, or acute distension of the stomach and small intestine. Ileus is a feature, and nasal reflux may also be seen. Subacute cases last for as long as one week.

Chronic cases, lasting as long as four weeks, are marked by depression, anorexia, drooling, and an increased heart rate. Droppings may be sparse or absent and, on rectal examination, the bowel may be empty, dry and mucus coated. There is marked weight loss, constipation and bowel stasis. Death may result from rupture of the bowel, followed by peritonitis. The pathologic lesion is found in the autonomic nervous system.

Treatment

There is no specific treatment for grass sickness, although symptomatic treatment may help some chronic animals to survive the disease. This includes fluid and electrolyte replacement, intravenous feeding, release of gas in the stomach through a stomach tube, and the promotion of normal bowel movement.

The treatment period may be long and expensive. It is important that those animals that do not respond quickly, and are suffering, should be humanely put out of their pain.

It has long been suggested that grass sickness may well be restricted to certain paddocks, during periods of lush grass growth. This being the case, it is wise to graze these paddocks with sheep or cattle at times of greatest risk. However, experience may show that the condition can occur in other circumstances.

Laminitis

Although the classical symptoms of laminitis are expressed in changes involving the laminae of the foot, the underlying problem frequently arises in the gut, and absorption of toxins is considered to be one of the prime causes. There is a distinct possibility of association with alterations in the natural gut bacterial flora, arising from changes in food constituents or from feeding procedures that disturb the balance of organisms.

Laminitis in ponies is more common because of a fundamental difference in metabolic processes between ponies and horses, the efficiency of food usage and fat storage.

The lesson to be learned from this condition, is that the anticipation of digestive upset is important and that the maintenance of bowel stasis should always be considered at times of risk. Risk not only includes dietary change but also stress caused in travel, competition, disease and its treatment, and like activities.

The use of probiotics may help to prevent sequelae of the nature of laminitis at times when dietary change is inevitable. Treatment of laminitis should always consider the removal of toxins – and toxin-producing organisms – from the gut, and re-establishment of a normal flora of organisms.

The local developments in the horse's feet may need to be treated as a specific pathology of those parts, although, if the primary cause is not treated, the condition can recur.

Cancer

The most common cancerous condition involving the bowel of the horse is lymphosarcoma, although other malignant tumours can occur. These include lipomas (involving fatty tissue) that are mostly seen in older horses and can be responsible for a type of strangulation of the gut that is not easily distinguished from other acute catastrophic types of colic.

Hernia

Abdominal hernias occur through natural or acquired openings in the abdominal wall, and are marked by the presence there of loops of bowel, or other abdominal contents.

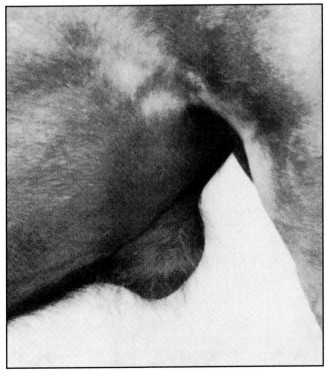

A horse with abdominal hernia

The most common hernias are in the umbilical and inguinal areas, and the possibility always exists that segments of bowel within the hernia will lose their blood supply and become strangulated.

Hernias of the abdominal musculature arise for reasons such as rupture of the prepubic tendon, and the greatest risk arises when this occurs in pregnant mares and the gravid uterus descends through lack of support.

Rupture of the diaphragm may allow the herniation of abdominal organs into the chest cavity, but this is a rare, and usually fatal, condition.

Nutritional causes of intestinal disease include over-feeding or the accidental access to food, mouldy feeds, and feeding irritants; also in this category will be sudden changes and disturbance of bacterial digestion by feeding too much grain and not enough fibre.

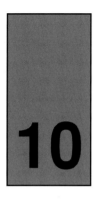

10 Infectious Diseases

Infectious diseases of the digestive system are caused by a number of recognised bacteria and viruses (also parasites; see Chapter 11), the most significant of which are *Salmonella* and Rotavirus, respectively. However, the extent and variety of potential pathogens is limitless and our knowledge of why they occur, how they cause disease, and what is the best way to treat them, is still developing.

Diarrhoea is a common expression of infectious digestive disease. However, although it can occur due to many other causes, it is included here because to discuss digestive infection without any understanding of diarrhoea would be pointless.

Diarrhoea

The occurrence of diarrhoea is mainly as a result of disturbed fluid and ion transport across the lining of the small or large intestine. Fluid that would normally be absorbed back into the system is retained within the gut and then passed out in the faeces. Frequently, the precipitating factor not being resolved, this fluid loss continues, or increases, with developing tissue reactions. The consequence is a very serious crisis for the animal's whole body, with massive fluid loss and inevitable death if the fluid loss cannot be dealt with. Abnormal gut motility can occur as a complication.

Loss of fluid occurs either because of failure of absorption or because of excessive secretion. Large amounts of fluid circulate between the blood and intestinal lumen, under normal circumstances greatly exceeding the daily fluid intake and amounting to a major proportion of the total body water. For example, a 100kg pony will absorb about 30 litres daily from the proximal small bowel.

These fluids include salivary, gastric, biliary and pancreatic secretions, all arising from extracellular fluid (ECF) and must therefore be proportionally reabsorbed to maintain blood and ECF volume. Thus, malabsorption of ions and water will lead to considerable fluid loss without any hypersecretion. This loss may result from virus-induced damage to the mucosa, or from invading bacteria. Hypersecretion occurs as a result of colonisation with toxin producing bacteria, even though the mucosa may appear normal. It can also appear with structural damage, as in *Salmonella*, or as a response to parasite infestation.

Diarrhoea is now considered to be a sign of dysfunction of the colon in the horse, even where the most prominent sign of the underlying disease is in the small intestine. The problem arises from the arrival in the colon of large amounts of improperly digested small intestine contents. The colon (and its resident organisms) is unable to deal with these and the consequence is the loss from the body of quantites of fluid which would otherwise be absorbed, as well as the loss of nutritive material required for growth and energy production.

Diarrhoea is a common problem of foals, less so in adult horses.

Clinical Signs

Affected animals may be tucked-up and seem to be dry or constipated before diarrhoea appears. Foul-smelling faeces may indicate putrefaction, tissue destruction, or simply reflect the diet. The colour of faeces in foal diarrhoea, as well as the consistency, can be an indication of the cause and severity of the condition. The presence of blood is always significant. Foals on milk, only, have yellow faeces but this changes as they eat grass, hay or solids.

While, inevitably, the primary sign of diarrhoea is excessively fluid faeces, the general condition of the animal is critical to treatment and to differential diagnosis. The presence, or absence, of a temperature is important, and elevated temperatures are generally an indication of systemic involvement. This could mean bacteria in the bloodstream, or absorbed toxins released from bacteria.

Anorexia is a common consequence of systemic infection, and is also particularly significant in foals, where a failure to suck is a very worrying development. Depression is a feature of some foal scours, and weight loss and lassitude may ensue.

In adults, sudden onset diarrhoea may be very acute and is frequently fatal. This type of condition is most often seen when there are major changes in the diet, or on moving from bare to rich pastures. Depression is common; temperatures may be elevated, but animals that have suffered acute fluid loss and are toxic may well have lower than normal temperatures.

Acute toxic enteritis occurs sporadically in older horses and symptoms include fever, depression, injected membranes, and often laminitis. There are numerous causes, *Salmonella*, *Clostridium*, antibiotic, NSAID, and colitis X among them. In many cases the primary cause is not identified; the most significant factor being inflammation of the tract with absorption of endotoxins. However, horses may have severe enteritis, dehydration and endotoxaemia without any diarrhoea.

Diagnosis

Finding the underlying cause of diarrhoea is critical to its treatment, as is deciphering the nature of the damage suffered by the bowel. Should it be caused by a virulent bacterial or viral infection, quick identification of the cause is necessary in order to stem spread and initiate treatment; equally, a sudden intake of parasite larvae would have implications for treatment.

Faecal swabs are submitted for laboratory examination in all cases that do not respond to immediate treatment or in situations where many animals are at risk. The offending organism is identified and sensitivity tests are carried out in the case of bacterial infection. An ELISA blood test for rotavirus infection is available.

If the problem is associated with dietary change, the animal's history may indicate this and appropriate measures may soon resolve the problem. Gross appearances of the faeces may reveal undigested material. Large quantities of mucus are an indication that the gut is inflamed, while blood (be it fresh, emanating from posterior parts of the tract; or dark, coming from the small bowel), perhaps, indicates a further progression of the disease.

Treatment

Certain priorities are basic to the treatment of diarrhoea. First, is to stem the immediate and ongoing fluid loss and replace that which has already been lost. It may well be that antibiotics are ineffective and that the provision of mechanical protection for damaged bowel with something like activated charcoal will help. Probiotics help to restore balance to the bowel flora of organisms. Fluid and electrolyte losses are restored by the administration of oral electrolyte solutions and in many cases this adequately resolves the loss, avoiding the need for intravenous fluid therapy.

The use of plasma, which may be primed to provide protection against a specific infection (like rotavirus), is often vital.

If the diarrhoea results from bacterial infection and endotoxaemia, there may be massive fluid loss and shock. Toxaemia may well lead to early death, but would require intensive intravenous treatment were the animal to survive.

Should the condition result from a sudden intake of parasite larvae, removal of these from the body would be a concern, when they became accessible to treatment. However, the immediate condition might call for fluid and electrolyte replacement in order to stem the loss of body condition.

Some 10–15 litres of plasma can be given to adults with diarrhoea and is considered beneficial. It is vital to give isotonic rather than hypertonic electrolyte solutions, in order to avoid further fluid loss.

Bismuth may be useful in adult horses. Drugs such as loperamide are capable of reducing fluid loss and increasing absorption. Activated charcoal is thought to absorb intraluminal toxins.

The primary cause of death in mature horses with diarrhoea is fluid and electrolyte imbalance or endotoxaemia. While antibiotic use is sometimes ineffective, when fluid levels have been restored, and a regular intake of replacement organisms is being given, the animal may benefit from injection with B vitamins.

It is important to maintain appetitie, as long as the intake of food does not risk further aggravating the condition. Inflamed tissues need to repair, and may need relative rest to achieve this. If the animal isn't eating (or a foal not drinking) liquid replacement with included electrolytes may provide this rest and maintain bodyweight. However, if the condition is prolonged, an energy source will be required, and intravenous therapy may be the only choice. In animals that will eat, without complication, the problem is less critical.

Endotoxaemia

Free endotoxin is present in the lumen of the bowel, a natural product in the turnover of gut bacteria. It is not normally absorbed in healthy bowel; however, disease can lead to degeneration of the bowel lining, letting endotoxin gain access to the peritoneal cavity and the circulation.

Endotoxin is a complex component of the outer cell wall of many gram-negative bacteria (endotoxaemia is the presence of these toxins within the vascular system). The intestinal bacterial flora constitutes a large reservoir of endotoxin, released without harm when bacteria die or undergo rapid growth.

When administered to horses in small doses endotoxin affects gut motility; but, in large doses, could cause death. Massive hypersecretion from the intestinal mucosa can cause rapid dehydration and death, possible side-effects of the inflammatory response to endotoxaemia.

Endotoxaemia is a feature of conditions like colitis X, many bacterial infections, and can occur in colic, even as a complication of meconium impaction of foals.

Clinical Signs

The clinical consequences of endotoxaemia are fever, a reduction of white blood cells, and a form of circulatory shock due to substantial fluid loss into the bowel, and diarrhoea. There is multiple organ failure and death. Depression is common, recumbency, congested membranes, dehydration, weak pulse, cold extremities, sweating, muscle tremors, all may be present.

Small haemorrhages may occur on mucous membranes, and laminitis may be a feature in less acute cases. Oedematous swellings on the abdomen may be seen in longer standing cases.

Diagnosis

The diagnosis will depend on clinical signs and on supportive blood analysis. The movement of fluid out of the circulation will be marked by a rise in packed cell volume (PCV), changes in serum proteins and acid base balance.

Treatment

Treatment involves intravenous use of blood expanders; plasma may be used, if cross-matched. NSAIDs (for example, flunixin) are used in treatment and prevention. A commercial antitoxin is now on the market and may prove a considerable help where the condition occurs.

The use of glucose and electrolyte solutions (given orally) to rehydrate animals suffering diarrhoea presumes absorption from the small intestine is still functional, but they do not stop the diarrhoea. Intravenous fluid is an alternative as, where there is malabsorption, the provision of oral solutions may only make matters worse.

Salmonella

At its most dangerous when infecting young foals, in which the disease varies from mild enteritis to severe bowel inflammation and septicaemia, *Salmonella* may prove fatal.

Salmonella organisms (of which over 2,000 serotypes have now been identified as causing disease in human beings) adhere to and invade the lining cells of the gut, resulting in an inflammatory response.

The source of the organism is usually an older horse; in intensive stud farms, it may be introduced by visiting stock. About 10 per cent of horses are considered to be *Salmonella* shedders and the dam may be the source of infection for a foal, the organism being picked up through faecal contamination of the environment.

Important factors are exposure dose, virulence of the bacterium, immune status, and stress. Stress is most likely to be a factor in adult infection and this may have led to a change of normal gut flora prior to infection, allowing *Salmonella* the opportunity to colonise.

Salmonella organisms produce endotoxins that increase permeability of the lining cells, stimulate secretion of water and electrolytes, and are capable of setting up severe systemic effects.

Clinical Signs

In adults, *Salmonella* can cause a number of types of disease from the acute to chronic diarrhoea. The source may be from any shedding animal; and a contaminated environment may remain thus for a long time. For example, soil may remain infective for 300 days, dried faeces for as long as 30 months, and water for 9 months. The organism survives freezing, but usually does not multiply outside a host. Drying and exposure to sunlight kill it.

In order for infection to occur, there needs to be an adequate dose of organism and this cannot be taken in over an indefinite period. Stress is an important precipitating factor. Stress may include exhaustion, change of diet, weaning, pregnancy, bad weather, transport, change from one farm to another, anaesthesia, surgery, antibiotic therapy and so on.

A change in the horse's intestinal flora probably plays a major role in development of the disease, the normal flora of the large intestine being hostile to *Salmonella*.

The early symptoms are depression, fever and anorexia, followed by abdominal pain within 24–48 hours. Diarrhoea occurs after about 48 hours, but may appear sooner or be delayed for as long as a week. Faeces have a foul smell and become progressively more watery once they start to be passed.

There may be a blue toxic ring on the gums, but horses that are alert and continue to eat have the best chance of recovering. In-foal mares may abort.

Salmonella is primarily an intracellular pathogen, meaning it lives within the host's cells, thus making it resistant to treatment. Diarrhoea may last three to four weeks and weight loss is severe in chronic cases.

Diagnosis

Specific diagnosis is made through faecal culture and identification of the organism in a laboratory. Negative results, however, are not necessarily conclusive.

Carriers should be detected by faecal culture and eliminated from a herd, although this is only possible if the organism is being passed and not if the animal is in a latent (not shedding) state. Five clear cultures at weekly intervals suggest an animal may no longer be a shedder. Most horses do not shed for more than eight weeks after recovery, but 10 per cent shed for a year or more.

Management is the most important factor in control. Endemic premises are those where large numbers of horses congregate – including race-tracks constructed in the style seen in the United States where horses live in barns on site. Salmonellosis occurs in high-density housing and when horses are placed under various stresses. Animals in transit should not be mixed with residents and movement of human contacts and equipment needs to be strictly controlled to limit infection. It is important to make no diet changes, to be careful about worm therapy, or other stresses, including vaccination. Good hygiene is an essential to prevent further spread.

Treatment

Antibiotics of the nature of chloramphenical, trimethoprim and ampicillin are sometimes effective, but the problem of treatment is hampered by the intracellular existance of the organism, and some authorities do not advise the use of antibiotics in this disease. Some of the more effective antibiotics have toxic side-effects, or are not considered due to expense.

Antibiotics may help if there is a septicaemia, but there is considerable resistance with this organism. Bismuth or activated charcoal may be helpful in protecting the inflamed bowel, reducing pain and reducing fluid loss. Plasma, especially from recovered adult animals, might be helpful, and flunixin may assist in reducing pain and countering toxaemia. It has been reported that horses on oral and parenteral antibiotics are 40 times more likely to get clinical salmonellosis than those that are not. This suggests that the antibiotic interferes with the normal gut flora and allows overgrowth by *Salmonella* species.

Fluid replacement is vital in therapy. Probiotics are a logical form of therapy, but, in so much as they support the normal flora, they are also useful in preventing the disease. Infection in foals that survive the immediate condition can be chronic and last for weeks.

The quality of management is what decides the incidence of *Salmonella* infection. Breeding stock should be kept separate from racing and performing animals to limit exposure to the bacterium.

Botulism

Caused by toxins of the bacterium, *Clostridium botulinum*, botulism is a disease of the nervous system, with paralysis. There are eight distinct toxin types, although symptoms are similar in each case.

Botulism occurs because of ingestion of preformed toxin or because of toxin production in damaged areas of bowel, or in wounds. Being an anaerobic organism, *C. botulinum* needs tissue damage to set up the proper conditions for growth. It will therefore not occur on hay, unless the hay is contaminated by rat carcasses or their like.

Most modern sources implicate silage or excessively moist hay, but the infection could also occur from ponds or water sources contaminated by dead animals.

Clinical Signs

The predominant sign of botulism is a progressive flaccid paralysis, occurring within 14 days of exposure to the source and exhibiting weakness and tremor of the limbs. This paralysis may progress from hindlimbs to forelimbs and eventually involve the jaw and throat, with paralysis of the tongue, inability to eat and the animal may roar. The large muscles of the forelimb may be affected, as also may those of the eyelids. Affected animals may be recumbent and unable to rise. Paralysis of the respiratory muscles may result in abdominal breathing.

There is incoordination, knuckling of the joints and ataxia. Sensation and consciousness remain until death. The tongue and tail are typically weak when subjected to manipulation.

Diagnosis

The signs are typical of the disease and will strongly suggest a diagnosis on their own. However, confirmation will depend on toxin identification in serum, liver, faeces or food sources. The organism may be cultured from faeces, although this might not be diagnostic in an adult animal.

Treatment

Antitoxin is available but will not affect toxin already bound to nervous tissue. Large doses, given intramuscularly, will neutralise circulating toxin, but the expense is considerable.

Supportive care is critical in animals with a chance of survival. Purgatives are given to clean toxins from the gut, and horses that cannot swallow must be fed and watered by stomach tube. Those that become recumbent are supported in slings; alternatively placed on thick bedding and rotated regularly. Ease of breathing must be assured and any form of exercise is not advisable.

Most horses with this condition cannot swallow on their own for as long as two weeks. Muzzling may help to prevent aspiration pneumonia. When recovery is anticipated, soft mashes are provided that are easily swallowed.

Prevention involves the use of antitoxin where animals are at risk of being exposed – or vaccination is common in endemic areas of the United States. Care should be taken when feeding silage that there is no chance of contamination. Other feed materials should be dry and not contain rodent carcasses. Carcasses of affected animals should be burned or buried deep in a well-drained area.

Intestinal Clostridiosis

Caused by *Clostridium perfringens* type A, intestinal clostridiosis is hard to distinguish from colitis X. There is a higher survival rate and a longer clinical course. The mortality rate is about 40 per cent.

Certain conditions (antibiotic use is one) may lead to raised levels of *C. pefringens* in the gut, but this has not been proven to be associated with disease. Clostridial organisms may be cultured from the gut of healthy animals; what turns this situation into disease is likely to involve a replacement of the normal flora with that of the disease-producing bacteria.

Clinical Signs

The condition is acute with depression and early diarrhoea. Death occurs in 12 hours to two days after illness commences. Recovery, if it occurs, is quick and dramatic.

At post-mortem there is acute colitis (inflammation of the colon). Lesions may also be found in the liver, kidneys and heart.

Diagnosis

Diagnosis depends on the isolation of larger than normal numbers of clostridia in faeces or intestinal contents. The presence of clostridial toxins in the bowel is not easily detectable and not available as a routine test from laboratories.

Treatment

Sour milk, containing lactose-utilising streptococci, has been found to be very effective, as should other forms of probiotic.

Colitis X

Colitis X is an acute disease of horses marked by profuse diarrhoea and a high mortality rate. Death usually occurs in the first 24 hours after symptoms appear. An associated stress is usually reported, be that a sudden change of diet or environment; a diet rich in protein and low in fibre is a common feature.

Horses of all ages are affected and the disease can occur at any time of the year. It is sporadic in occurrence, except at USA-style racetracks where it may become endemic. In the United Kingdom and in Ireland it is seen on stud farms as a sporadic disease, and is not uncommon when horses are moved from poor to rich pastures.

Clinical Signs

Affected horses are very sick. They will have high temperatures, injected membranes, signs of acute dehydration, shock and severe depression.

The abdomen may be distended, with no sign of diarrhoea, or there may be severe diarrhoea. The pulse is weak, mucous membranes are dry, and there is an increased heart rate. Diarrhoea, when it occurs, comes in large volume, and is watery and smelly. There is shock, consequent on the loss of huge volumes of fluid and absorption of endotoxins.

Few horses survive this condition and post-mortem lesions are found in the caecum and colon which may show severe inflammation. There are no changes in the stomach, ileum, duodenum, or jejunum. The lungs may show oedema and emphysema.

Diagnosis

The cause of colitis X is unknown although there is a recent suggestion that it might be due to *Clostridium perfringens* type A endotoxaemia. There may be confusion with other forms of acute diarrhoea (like *Salmonella*), but the diagnosis will be suggested by the nature of the condition and the post-mortem findings.

Treatment

Treatment is seldom successful but consists of fluid replacement therapy, which may require as much as 20 litres per hour as well as drugs to fight toxaemia and shock. Horses that survive two days have a chance of recovery.

Rotavirus

Rotavirus is discussed in more detail as a disease of foals (see Chapter 12.) Almost 100 per cent of adult horses have antibodies and 30 per cent of foals with diarrhoea have had Rotavirus identified; yet, the true role of the virus in infection is not fully understood.

The disease occurs as an epidemic, in most outbreaks, and the source of infection may be adult shedders. Foals, mainly, show signs of infection; and while mares provide some protection in their milk this does not prevent infection where there is a heavy challenge.

Rotavirus infection is a major cause of disruption to stud farms, and outbreaks may be very time consuming to deal with. Recumbent foals, perhaps in large numbers, may have to be sustained by fluid therapy, and losses are not uncommon.

Other Viruses

Coronavirus has been associated with diarrhoea in foals, a rate of 15 per cent mortality attributed to it and 40 per cent morbidity. There is a sudden outbreak of profuse watery diarrhoea with a febrile response.

Adenovirus has been retrieved from immune-normal foals suffering diarrhoea. It is not thought to be a primary pathogen, though it may act as a secondary organism in some situations.

Potomac Horse Fever

Caused by *Ehrlichia risticii*, an intracellular parasite, Potomac fever is known as equine diarrhoeal syndrome. The clinical signs result from inflammation of the small intestine and the colon.

Potomac fever occurs all over the United States, mostly in endemic areas. The condition is seasonal with first cases appearing sporadically in the late spring and the last in the autumn, maybe one or two cases per farm. Contact with recovered or sick animals is not necessary, and horses of all ages and types are affected.

It is assumed that there is a fly vector (though this is not proven) and a mechanism for over-wintering of the organism must exist.

Clinically, there is anorexia, depression and fever. There may be abdominal pain and diarrhoea, and laminitis may be seen as an initial symptom. Some animals show a blue ring on the gums at initial examination and the membranes are injected. There may be no abdominal sounds and fluid is detected in the gut. Heart and respiratory rates are increased. Dehydration is a common feature, although 40 per cent of horses do not have diarrhoea.

Symptoms are typical of acute toxic colitis of any other source. Serology is used in diagnosis, but there may be difficulty in establishing the cause.

Treatment is with fluid therapy and specific antibiotics are used against the causal organism, though these need to be selected with care if the diagnosis is not established. The mortality rate is up to 30 per cent, this often being influenced by post-infection laminitis.

Diarrhoea Caused by Antibiotics

Fatal colitis has resulted from feeding lincomycin, tylosin, erythromycin, tetracycline and neomycin, also trimethoprim/sulfa drugs, penicillin, metronidazole and cephalosporins.

The pathogenesis is not well understood, but the primary consequence is the over-growth of toxigenic bacteria, the identity of which is disputed. There may, too, be a synergistic effect between diet, environment and antibiotic.

Oral use of drugs is most likely to cause the problem.

The most serious pathogens in the condition are *Salmonella* species and *Clostridium perfringens*.

Clinical Signs

Within two to five days of exposure to the antibiotic signs usually appear. There is profuse watery diarrhoea, anorexia and lethargy. Colic may occur in time, increased heart rate, injected membranes and fever. Badly affected animals die in three to five days, though the condition may be mild in nature.

There is shock and dehydration detected on blood analysis. Post-mortem findings are of an enlarged and oedematous colon filled with serosanguinous (blood and serum) fluid; there is also haemorrhage into the kidneys. Clotting may be delayed and there may be diffuse small haemorrhages on visceral organs.

Surviving horses may develop laminitis.

Diagnosis

Diagnosis depends on the history of antibiotic use with the development of diarrhoea.

Treatment

There is no specific antidote to diarrhoea, but the most logical approach to the condition is to replace lost fluid and attempt to re-establish the normal gut flora by using probiotics. Activated charcoal and mineral oil may be useful to prevent further absorption of toxins. Fluid therapy needs to be aggressive. Rest and supportive care are needed to prevent a relapse.

Diarrhoea Caused by Other Organisms

Sometimes, *Rhodococcus equi* (discussed later in more detail as a disease of foals in Chapter 12) causes diarrhoea in adults. It may be associated with abscesses in the lymph nodes of the gut or with diffuse colitis. Presence of the organism in the faeces is not diagnostic. Erythromycin and rifampin are the antibiotics of choice.

Escherichia coli is not considered a significant cause of diarrhoea in horses. The horse does not appear sensitive to *E. coli* endotoxins.

Although *Campylobacter* has been implicated in foal diarrhoea with temperature, colic, acute diarrhoea and ulcer formation, findings are not conclusive. Treatment would involve identification of the organism and use of an antibiotic based on sensitivity tests.

Another possible cause of bacterial diarrhoea is *Streptococcus* species. It is conceivable that a wide range of organisms is capable of invading the damaged or debilitated bowel. The primary cause is, therefore, the damaged tissue, not the presence of organisms, and infection may ensue from any organism that is present to exploit the situation. The first principle of treatment has to be the restoration of tissue health, the replacement of lost fluids, and the re-establishment of a normal gut flora.

Fungal colitis may be caused by *Aspergillus* or *Mucor* species. There is high temperature and sudden development of diarrhoea. Peritonitis can occur and symptoms tend to be very severe. The condition is usually diagnosed post-mortem, and may be associated with antibiotic therapy. Symptoms are similar to those of colitis X except horses live for up to 48 hours.

Peritonitis

Infection of the peritoneum is the possible result of parasite migration, abscess rupture or intestinal perforation. Many cases recover and the cause is unknown, but the condition can be extremely serious and lead to death.

Abdominal pain is a feature, and the animal may stand rigidly with a tense and tender abdomen; it is unlikely to lie down. Anorexia, elevated temperature and injected membranes are seen. Diarrhoea may also be a symptom, although constipation may alternatively occur. Diagnosis should be confirmed on paracentesis and blood analysis will show alterations in the white blood cells resulting from infection.

It is important in considering treatment to know the underlying cause. If there is leakage from the bowel, broad-spectrum antibiotics are used, but it must be ensured these reach the affected area in adequate concentrations to be effective. Fluid therapy may be necessary, especially to ensure there is adequate energy if the animal refuses to eat.

Where the condition is due to abscess formation, *R. equi* could be involved, or migrating larvae, and the choice of drugs will depend on the organism. Diffuse peritonitis can localise and form abscesses or adhesions, though this is rare. Adhesions may be extensive in the aftermath of this condition, providing a poor prognosis.

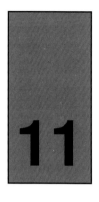

11 Parasites of the Digestive System

The influence of parasitic diseases on the bowel is extensive and is due to a number of factors relating to the nature and life-cycles of the parasites themselves as well as the ways in which they achieve their often complex manoeuverings within the animal host. This influence is further complicated by the possibility of multiple parasite infestation in many, if not most, situations.

Some of the ways in which this influence occurs are discussed in this chapter. The discussion is in alphabetical order, rather than in any order of importance.

Absorption

It is natural to expect that where there is extensive damage to the bowel lining, absorption will be affected. In this event, food material may pass along the bowel undigested, leading to further complications, including fluid loss and diarrhoea in some cases.

Problems associated with malabsorption, as already discussed (see Chapter 9), are capable of affecting other body systems, like blood and bone.

Allergic Reactions

The occurrence of allergic reactions is dependent on the complex interactions between host tissues and the parasite, its tissues, or excretions. The extent of these reactions can be very considerable and greatly exacerbate the disease process. This is most serious in young animals where a gradual intake of worms allows the development of such immune-related reactions.

Anaemia

A common feature of parasite disease, anaemia results from the blood-sucking habits of worms such as members of the strongyle family, also liver fluke, and the like. It can also result from bleeding due to tissue tearing by worms, or from failure to absorb constituents essential to the formation of blood.

Aneurysms

Digestive tract disease in horses is marked by the influence of worm induced aneurysms that cut off blood supply and produce types of colic that are frequently fatal. The aneurysms are formed by the larval stages of parasites that migrate to sites within blood vessels. When released in clumps they form emboli that sometimes deprive bowel sections of blood.

Anorexia

With heavy worm infestations, foals, especially, may go off their food and lose weight.

The cause of the anorexia is thought in some cases to result from parasite effects on digestion. This problem may be exacerbated where the parasite is in direct competition with the host for food material within the bowel. Anorexia may also result from pain caused by worm migrations or to disturbances of metabolism due to infestation.

Diarrhoea

A common consequence of heavy worm burdens, especially in younger animals, is diarrhoea. As already suggested, this may result from digestive failure as much as other influences of the parasite. Its consequence is dehydration and weight loss.

Mechanical Obstruction

The horse roundworm, *Parascaris,* may be present in such large numbers, especially in the bowel of foals, that it physically obstructs the passage of food.

Parascaris worms may also, at times, block the bile ducts. Should this happen, the animal may show evidence of jaundice.

Physical Injury

Parasites, in both their larval and mature stages, damage surface tissues of the bowel by tearing and blood-sucking. The extent of such damage may be considerable, especially depending on the degree of infestation suffered by the animal.

Immature stages of the small redworm, *Cyathostomum*, develop within the wall of the bowel, causing local tissue damage, leading to general areas of inflammation, and, perhaps, ulceration. Naturally, too, the production of digestive enzymes, and the like, will also be affected.

This aspect of infestation can lead to considerable pain, which will cause further influence on bodyweight and development.

Protein Loss

The amount of protein in the gut may be increased in parasitic disease because of failure of absorption as well as protein loss as a result of tissue damage and effusion of serum and plasma into the lumen. The end result of this may be weight loss and oedema.

Worm Types

One of the primary effects of worm infestation is, therefore, disease of the digestive system. There are various varieties of worm, some of which are discussed in the following pages.

Roundworms

Any worm type of the class *Nematoda* is known as a roundworm. These are commonly a cause of infestation in horses and have a considerable health and economic importance.

The worms are noted for the possession of a digestive tract and, in the case of strongyles, mouthparts adapted for biting tissues, with which they are capable of doing extensive damage. These worms are 'plug-feeders', that is, they bite off plugs of surface material from the host's intestine as they feed. They also are a common cause of anaemia through direct and indirect blood loss.

The life-cycle of strongyles means that laying females shed eggs into the grazing environment, through which other horses become infected. These eggs may then develop through larval stages before being ingested by the new host (or, as in the case of *Parascaris*, are ingested as larva-containing eggs, to develop within the host). Generally, maturation occurs and the adult female produces her eggs in the bowel. These eggs are passed in the faeces.

Large Strongyles

The large redworms (named by the colour they acquire through sucking blood), *Strongylus vulgaris*, *S. equinus* and *S. edentatus*, are especially significant here because their larvae penetrate the bowel wall and migrate through blood vessels, where the prospect of aneurysm formation arises, with all the possible complications that can engender for the host. Adults have strong-coated stout bodies that measure between 2–5cm in length.

Thankfully, as a better family of drugs has emerged to deal with larval redworms, the incidence of acute colic, caused by emboli (clumps) of immature worms blocking off blood supply to bowel segments, has become significantly reduced.

The migratory phases of some of these worms also take them through organs like the liver, where their influence may ultimately have other adverse effects on the digestive system. The location of the mature worm is the large intestine, including the caecum. Redworms have a clinical presence wherever horses are kept. They cause protein as well as blood loss, disturb fluid balance and provoke diarrhoea. Peritonitis is another possible effect.

Typical redworm egg

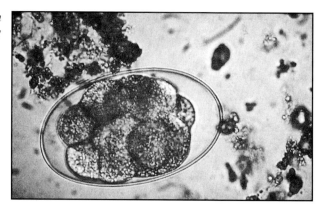

Adult large redworms in bowel

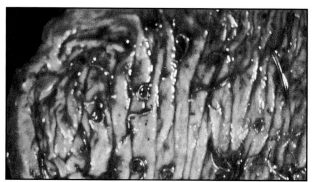

Diagnosis is through the identification of strongyle eggs in faeces, or by direct identification of adult worms post-mortem.

Small Strongyles

Today, of the eight different families of small strongyle, *Cyathostomum* species are the most significant entity clinically.

These worms measure only between 5–25mm in length, but they are marked by huge populations that can build up within a host (as many as a million worms have been found in an individual animal). During development within the host, the worms become encysted in the wall of the host's large intestine and caecum. As they emerge from this site in the spring, small strongyles are responsible for inflammation of the colon, acute diarrhoea, and weight loss.

The problem has been compounded by a degree of resistance to the available anthelmintics (drugs that kill helminth parasites), especially when larvae are encysted.

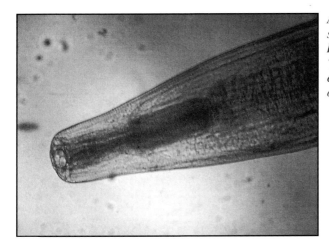

Anterior end of small redworm. Being a 'plug-feeder', this end tears out plugs of bowel wall

Small strongyles are also blood-sucking plug feeders. Large infestations can result in colic, emaciation and oedema. Diagnosis is made difficult when eggs are not found in faeces, the females producing only relatively small numbers of eggs. However, this may be offset by the presence of large numbers of larvae, which can then be identified.

Threadworm

The threadworm, *Strongyloides westeri*, is another roundworm, adults of which are most commonly found in suckling and weanling foals. The significance of this infection is gradually diminished as foals mature. Within the host, threadworms live deep in the lining of the intestine, especially the small intestine.

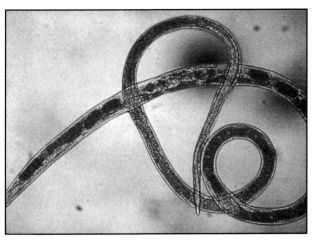

Adult threadworm

A significant feature of threadworm infection is the transmission of larvae from the mare to her foal through the milk. There is today some suggestion that such transmission may be a cause of foaling-heat scours, though this suggestion is disputed.

During their migratory stages, larvae visit the lungs, but then grow to maturity in the small intestine. *S. westeri* are capable of penetrating the skin.

Severe damage to the lining of the small intestine may occur in heavy infestations, with consequent disturbance of digestion. Diarrhoea is a symptom of infection in young animals.

Diagnosis is based on the presence of eggs and larvae in the faeces.

The Horse Roundworm

A large and frequently encountered parasite, *Parascaris equorum* is most commonly referred to as 'the horse roundworm'. Adults grow to as long as 50cm in length. Eggs from these worms are notably weather-resistant, and are ingested by the new host while containing a developing larva. When hatched, these larvae penetrate the wall of the small intestine and migrate via the blood and liver to the lungs. They climb the trachea before reaching the small intestine, where they grow to maturity. Females are prolific egg-layers and the eggs, which are sticky and may attach to a mare's udder, remain viable for years. *Parascaris* is a common cause of disease and is world-wide in distribution.

In foals, the symptoms of roundworm infestation include weight loss, poor coat and swollen abdomen. Clumps of mature worms may be so large they can virtually block the intestine. Allergic reactions to the presence of the worm may exacerbate clinical effects. Enteritis may result

The resistant eggs of horse roundworm

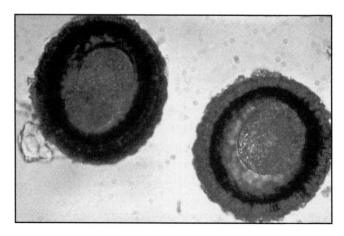

from the presence of this worm, marked by diarrhoea or constipation. Diagnosis is made by the presence of easily-recognised eggs in the faeces.

The Hairworm

About 0.5cm in length, *Trichostrongylus axei*, the hairworm parasitises the stomach glands and small intestine of the horse. As it also infects cattle and sheep, it is especially significant where there is mixed grazing.

The hairworm exists in most temperate countries and its larvae are durable and capable of surviving through the winter.

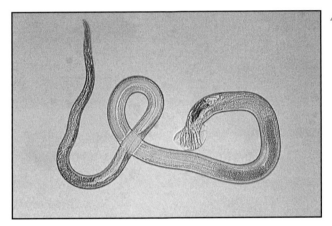

Adult hairworm

The presence of this worm irritates the stomach lining, resulting in plaque formation, erosion of the surface tissues and blood loss. There is anaemia, protein depletion and diarrhoea. Affected animals lose weight and may become oedematous.

Identification is not made on the basis of finding eggs in faeces, but depends on larval culture.

The Pinworm

A plug-feeder in its larval stages, *Oxyuris equi*, the pinworm, is capable of causing considerable damage to the bowel. Adults, the female of which are often 10cm long, feed only on intestinal contents.

The female lays her eggs in sticky clumps on the skin of the perinaeum around the host's anus. These clumps detach in flakes to contaminate the stable area or ground. Ingested larvae penetrate the wall of the large intestine, from which area mature females move to the anus for egg-laying.

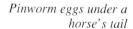

*Pinworm eggs under a
horse's tail*

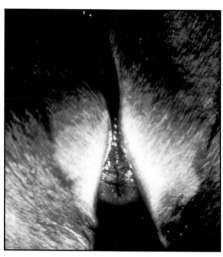

The eggs in the anal area irritate the horse and cause scratching which may lead to self-mutilation. Lesions in the large intestine may ulcerate and affected animals lose weight, may be anorexic and suffer anxiety.

The egg clumps under the tail are diagnostic and smears taken from these clumps will generally reveal large numbers of eggs which can be identified microscopically. Some affected horses will not scratch.

Abdominal Worm

Differing from the worms already discussed in this section, *Setaria equina*, the abdominal worm, produces microfilaria (embryonic larvae) instead of eggs. It is a parasite of horses in warm areas of the world and involves an intermediate host, a mosquito, that transmits the infection from horse to horse while feeding. The adult worms are parasites of serous membranes in the abdominal cavity, but may be found in other sites. They are not clinically very significant, although they may cause serious problems where they gain entry to an eye, or to the brain or spinal cord.

Stomach Worms

All stomach worms, *Habronema muscae*, *H. microstoma* and *Draschia megastoma* are the cause of cutaneous habronemiasis, or 'summer sores'.

Again, there is an intermediate host – the house fly being one – that picks up the larvae from faeces. These flies allow development of the larvae and eventually deposit them on the soft, moist tissues of the lips, nostrils and prepuce, or on wounds, from whence the horse licks and ingests them and they develop to maturity in the stomach.

Adult worms reside on the lining of the stomach under thick plugs of mucus. They do not cause great harm in this situation. *D. megastoma* causes the formation of nodules in the stomach that may develop into tumour-like growths which may become large enough to block entry of food into the small intestine. The growths, too, may well interfere with digestion if the worm is present in large numbers.

Diagnosis depends on the presence of eggs or larvae in faeces.

Gullet Worm

A parasite of the oesophagus, *Gongylonema pulchrum*, the gullet worm, can measure as much as 15cm in length, but is not considered significant as a cause of disease. Dung beetles act as the intermediate host.

Cestoda

The only cestodes (different class of worm from the *Nematoda*) to infest horses are the tapeworms, *Anoplocephala perfoliata* and *A. magna*. Adult parasites can be as much as 80cm long and 2cm wide. They consist of short segments (proglottids) which become enlarged with eggs and are released into the grazing environment in faeces. Tapeworms are thought to affect as many as 50 per cent of horses world-wide. The oribatid mite acts as an intermediate host, picking eggs up in faeces and then being eaten by horses when grazing.

Larvae grow to maturity in the lower small intestine, the caecum and

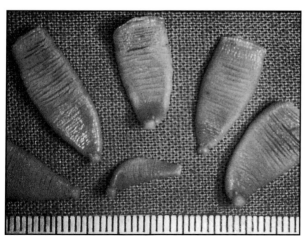

Adult tapeworms showing the scolex at the narrow end; the cross-stripes mark the division of the proglottids

Tapeworm eggs

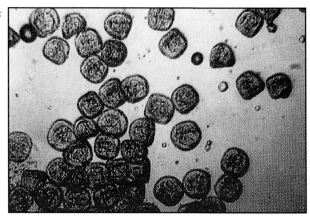

colon. Large worm burdens develop which cannot benefit the host, although there is some argument as to their clinical significance. Tapeworms compete with the host for food, and may also cause some irritation to the gut wall. Intestinal blockage may occur from the accumulation of tapeworms in the terminal small intestine.

Affected horses lose weight, may exhibit signs of colic, and can have persistent diarrhoea.

Although diagnosis depends on finding tapeworm segments or eggs in the faeces, there can be negative findings even in heavy infestations.

Liver Fluke

The most commonly found trematode (another class of worm) in horses is the liver fluke, *Fasciola hepatica*. Another is the lancet fluke, *Dicrocoelium dendriticum*, which occurs in parts of Europe. The intermediate host of the liver fluke is a freshwater snail. The parasite is

Liver fluke egg

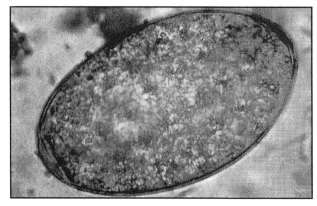

distributed on a world-wide basis in those areas where habitats suitable to the requirements of the snail are found. Eggs of adult fluke, which reside in the bile ducts, are carried to the intestine in the bile, from which they are passed to the exterior in faeces. Horses become infected by eating grass on the verges of the wet areas inhabited by the snail. Immature fluke migrate through the substance of the liver, interfering with normal liver function and causing acute tissue destruction, depending on the level of infection.

Affected horses are anaemic, lose weight and suffer digestive disturbances.

Diagnosis is not easily made and is dependent on finding eggs in the faeces.

The Botfly

Although the horse botfly, *Gasterophilus intestinalis*, has long been seen as a problem, the exact clinical significance of its infestation has been questioned.

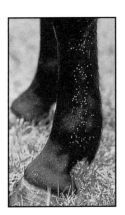
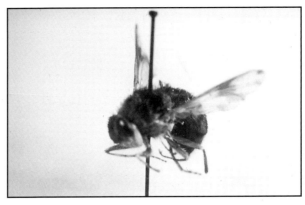

Bot eggs (left) *on a horse's leg; and* (right) *the adult botfly*

The flies lay eggs on horses' body and leg hair. The horses lick these eggs off and, subsequently, larvae hatch out and invade the horses' tongue, eventually moving to the stomach, where they over-winter.

Bots attach to the lining of the stomach, and are often present in large numbers. They may become so numerous as to physically interfere with digestion, or block the passage of food. The site of their attachment is marked by a deep ulcer around which the tissue is thickened. It has been known for bots to cause peritonitis by burrowing through the wall of the stomach.

The migrations of the larvae through the tongue and other tissues of the mouth can be very irritating and result in weight loss in heavily infected animals.

Bot eggs are easily recognised, seen as rows of small yellow dots that adhere firmly to the hair. Bot larvae are found in the faeces, some 2–3cm long, deep red, or yellow, in colour. They are often seen after dosing with an effective drug.

12 Digestive Diseases of the Foal

Newborn foals are protected by immunoglobulins (IG) in colostrum from infections they might encounter in early life. Protection is, effectively, against organisms the dam has encountered and will include many potential pathogens in the immediate environment. The foal is born without this spread of protection and also possesses a gut that is, to all intents and purposes, sterile. The foal, therefore, depends on the quality of the dam's milk for early immunity – and the natural flora of digestive organisms develops through contact with the environment.

Foals are totally dependent on colostrum for passive immunity after birth, there being no placental transfer during pregnancy. To be fully effective, this transfer must occur in the first 12–24 hours of life and may be impossible after this time. In fact, it is good practice to ensure the foal drinks from the mare within the first hour, as transfer of immunity may become less efficient as time elapses. Also, where a mare has run milk prior to foaling, the benefit to the foal can be seriously undermined, and might need to be supplemented by stored (or fresh) colostrum from another mare.

To provide information of the immune status, blood samples are taken when the foal is one day old. Foals with less than 400 mg/dl of serum IG need supplementation with plasma.

Colostrum for storage is best taken from newly-foaled mares that have a surplus of milk; this can then be frozen and held for future use. Between 2–4 litres of plasma, given intravenously, is necessary to protect foals that are without protection.

Immunodeficiency is a hereditary disease of Arabian foals, expressed as respiratory or digestive system infections. This is especially expressed in the case of adenovirus infection, which is usually fatal.

- If there is inadequate intake of colostrum
- If there are inadequate amounts of immunoglobin in the colostrum
- When there is early closure of the gut epithelium, before the foal has had time to suck.

Summary: the reasons for the failure of passive protection occurring in foals

Meconium Retention

Retained meconium (first faecal material of the newborn) is a problem of the first 48 hours of life although its influence seldom extends beyond this period. It is distinguished from infectious conditions by the lack of a temperature, dehydration, toxicity, and diarrhoea.

The retention of meconium is primarily a problem of colt foals. It is common in Thoroughbreds, and may become particularly troublesome in rare, isolated cases.

The problem is due to the formation of large faecal pellets that have difficulty traversing the colt's small pelvic canal. It is a simple matter of pellet oversize, usually, and nothing more sinister than that. More rarely, atresia ani (absence of normal opening of anus) is the cause of similar problems, but this is evident on inspection.

In many large studs, all colt foals are routinely given a phosphate enema as soon as they have sucked, as a preventive measure. Using the commercially-available human preparation, in a plastic container with a long, soft applicator, the fluid is introduced gently into the rectum, where it begins to work very quickly. Needless to say, the procedure must be undertaken with care and gentleness, as it is possible to do irreparable damage by using force on such delicate tissues. However, phosphate enemas are commonly administered by experienced grooms who will quickly seek veterinary help in complicated cases, and who will readily appreciate the risks involved.

Foals that are still unable to pass meconium display signs of colic of varying degrees, often rolling and pawing in pain. Acute cases show severe symptoms with sweating and it is vital that these animals are seen by a vet, who may decide to give mineral oil by stomach tube, or even sedatives, to ease the discomfort. However, it must be understood that meconium retention is a mechanical condition and, generally, if the foal is kept sucking, the developing pressure of digested material will relieve the problem. On rare occasions, surgery is needed to resolve the blockage.

Retained meconium is also sometimes associated with rupture of the bladder, with urine retention within the abdomen. Affected foals show abdominal distension and the problem is diagnosed by examination of collected abdominal fluid. Treatment is by surgery.

Foaling-heat Diarrhoea

A plethora of causes are suggested for foaling-heat diarrhoea, among which are hormonal changes affecting the dam and the early infection of foals with *Strongyloides westeri* parasites. In reality, the cause is still unknown, and there are also suggestions that it might be due to developmental changes in the digestive tract of the foal.

Diarrhoea occurs between the first 5–14 days of life; the foal generally is otherwise symptomless, with no temperature and continues to suck, a crucial factor in dealing with the condition.

When the only symptom is a milk-coloured diarrhoea, with no failure to suck, no temperature and no dehydration, the condition should be observed and no interference is advised. Where the amount and consistency of the faeces increases and becomes more fluid, activated charcoal may be given orally. Should signs of dehydration appear, like a dry coat, and/or loss of condition, electrolytes may have to be given orally, perhaps by stomach tube. There is generally no need for antibiotics, unless there is evidence of secondary bacterial involvement with systemic invasion. A more logical benefit might be had from the use of probiotics.

Salmonella

At its most dangerous when infecting young foals, *Salmonella* can prove fatal. The disease influence varies from mild enteritis to severe bowel inflammation and septicaemia. All foals with *Salmonella* are at risk of systemic infection, possibly leading to joint infection. For this reason infected foals, generally, should be treated with antibiotics.

The possible source of the infection is usually an older horse, although the risk is greatest in intensive stud farms where infection may be introduced from visiting stock. About 10 per cent of horses are considered to be *Salmonella* shedders and the dam may be the source of infection for a foal, the organism being picked up from the environment.

Important factors are exposure dose, virulence of the bacterium, immune status, and stress. Foals are more susceptible to *Salmonella* organisms because they are only developing their natural flora and because of their immature immune status. Weaning is a common time for cases to appear.

Clinical Signs

The foal may be depressed and off food for 24–48 hours before signs appear, although this may only be realised retrospectively. A suckling foal may be creating the impression it's sucking, though without vigour (easily noticed because the mare's udder becomes filled). There may be mild abdominal pain and a raised temperature.

Symptoms increase as time passes and abdominal distension can develop before diarrhoea – which is watery, foetid and profuse – starts.

Foals dehydrate even before diarrhoea is seen (because of fluid loss into the intestine) and have dry membranes and sunken eyes. Loud splashing sounds may be heard on palpating the abdomen, but no peristaltic sounds. Surface membranes are likely to be injected. Heart and respiratory rates are increased. Faeces will have a foul odour and there may be staining of the tail area. Swelling of the joints indicates septicaemic spread and meningitis may occur.

Treatment

As pointed out earlier (see Chapter 10), the treatment of *Salmonella* infections using antibiotics is often unsatisfactory because of the nature of the organism – and because of resistance – but antibiotic therapy is still a priority for foals.

Early diagnosis and treatment is important. The systemic effects of the infection have to be catered for, with fluid replacement, acid-base balance control, and so on. The condition within the bowel may be helped by bowel protectants like activated charcoal, and probiotic use may also be very beneficial.

Where fluid replacement becomes necessary, the equivalent of 20 per cent bodyweight per day is about what a normal foal would consume. If this is milk, or milk replacer, the total is given in hourly feeds to a very young foal, the time lapses increasing as the foal gets older. The amount to begin with, especially with a sick foal, might be as little as 5 per cent bodyweight per day, which will sustain life, and this may be increased as seen advisable, depending on the foal's ability to cope.

The foal has a small stomach and, for this reason, should not be given large, irregular feeds. Hourly, or bi-hourly, feeds are required during the first week of life and, as the foal gets stronger, this regime can be altered to suit both human and animal demands. Foals that cannot tolerate oral feeding may have to be fed intravenously.

Tyzzer's Disease

An acute bacterial infection of the liver, caused by *Bacillus piliformis*, this organism is thought to enter the body through ingestion.

Natural incidents of the infection are sporadic. Adult horses or rodents may act as reservoir hosts, though the condition could be an expression of reduced immunity.

Tyzzer's disease is highly fatal in foals aged between 7–42 days old, and affected foals may be found dead. A high fever is accompanied by depression and rapid coma development: there is severe hypoglycaemia. Foals that survive 24 hours show marked jaundice and nervous signs. Shock may be observed and subnormal temperatures are a feature of this disease.

On post-mortem examination, focal areas of necrosis (tissue death) are found in the liver which may be enlarged. Jaundice, petechiae (pinpoint haemorrhages) and areas of focal necrosis are also found on other organs. The organisms are seen on microscopic study of liver sections.

The prognosis is poor and treatment seldom is effective.

Necrotizing Enterocolitis

A disease marked by acute diarrhoea, faeces in necrotizing enterocolitis is often bloody in character. There may be colic-type pain, raised temperature and abdominal swelling. The cause of the condition is unknown, although *Clostridium perfringens* infection has been suggested, but is unlikely to be the only cause. Prematurity, stress and immune status have also been considered. Abdominal swelling is caused by excessive gas production within the bowel.

Foals suffering from necrotizing enterocolitis would have to be fed intravenously, until the bowel inflammation was alleviated. Antibiotics may also be used, given intravenously also.

Rhodococcus Equi

Formerly known as *Corynebacterium equi*, *Rhodococcus equi* causes pneumonia, most commonly, in foals on a world-wide basis and rarely in older horses. It is, too, sometimes the cause of diarrhoea in weanling foals.

Abscesses occur in the lymph nodes of the digestive system and invasion of the bowel wall may produce ulcers, which are associated with pain and diarrhoea. The organism is intracellular, growing within cells it invades and provoking the formation of thick-walled abscesses.

An incidence as high as 17 per cent in foals world-wide has been reported with a mortality rate of 80 per cent, although this incidence is not experienced in the United Kingdom and Ireland, except on some individual farms. Mortality is highest in foals about two months old but the condition can occur up to six months or more. Management and environmental factors play major roles in determining the magnitude of the challenge, and therefore affect the prevalance of the disease.

The ability of foals to withstand this infection is dependent on both the size of the challenge and the effectiveness of immune transfer from the dam. The organism is considered part of the normal gut flora, and foals may become infected by eating droppings (coprophagia). It is also present in soil, even in land not grazed by horses, and most likely to be encountered in the warmer months of the year.

The prevalence of infection increases with dusty environments and dry weather, and the organism is not affected by direct sunlight. Foals kept in stables may be more at risk of inhaling the organism than when at pasture, because of the special parameters of indoor environment.

The main routes of infection are the digestive and respiratory tracts. Ingestion rarely leads to respiratory disease; inhalation causes disease in the respiratory tract, especially the lungs. Once ingested, the organism penetrates the bowel and causes abscess formation in local lymph nodes. In the lungs, abscesses are formed in lymph nodes and in lung tissue.

Although infection is thought to occur in the neonatal period, signs are often not noticed until the foal is more than a month old.

Clinical Signs

Two clinical forms of *Rhodococcus equi* exist: subacute and chronic. In the subacute form foals die within days of showing respiratory distress. The lesions in these foals are chronic in nature although the disease is said to be subacute. In the chronic form, pneumonia and unthriftiness progress for weeks or months, and foals that survive may have permanently damaged lungs.

Some foals are found dead with lung abscesses located on postmortem. Other foals have high fever, rapid, deep breathing, and may be anxious, with discoloured membranes. They are usually off suck and weak, and may not lie down. Nasal discharge and coughing are inconsistent. Severely affected foals die within days despite treatment, but other cases have a more chronic course. These animals may have prolonged or recurrent fever, suffer depression, breathe heavily, lose condition and become unthrifty. Cough, if present, is usually soft and deep. Some have enlarged joints, with or without evident lameness.

Diagnosis

Haematology may reveal an increased white cell count, but this is not specific for R. equi infection. Radiography is used to identify lesions in the lungs. The organism can be isolated from material taken directly from lesions or from tracheal exudates. False negatives can occur due to the organism not growing on a culture medium. This occurs because the bacterium may be contained within defensive blood cells, therefore not within access of the growth medium. Results of ELISA tests have been variable. Other blood and antibody tests can be equally unsatisfactory.

Treatment

The organism responds to some antibiotics, although infections of this nature are naturally resistant (because the antibiotics cannot reach the infecting organism in high enough concentrations), and, even in successful cases, treatment may be very prolonged, and expensive. Plasma from the mare is used to good effect in early treatment and affected foals require nursing, adequate warmth and nourishment.

Fluid replacement is important where there is dehydration, and both carbohydrates and protein are provided in easily digested form to ensure they are absorbed from the small intestine.

To prevent this disease, foals should be housed in properly ventilated, but warm, dust-free areas. Dirt paddocks are best avoided, as are congested stable areas; dusty areas of pastures should be fenced off. When no other option exists, manure should be removed from infected paddocks, the paddocks to be rotated; otherwise all foals should be kept off endemic farms.

Sick foals are usually isolated; in contacts are examined two or three times a week, taking temperatures, examining the lungs, watching for diarrhoea. It is important to carry out post-mortem examinations on all dead foals.

Rotavirus Infection

A common cause of diarrhoea, Rotavirus infection occurs in foals from four days to five months of age. It can become endemic on stud farms and affect a very high percentage of foals.

The infection itself is sometimes mild in character, although usually not lethal, except where secondary bacterial infections become established, or in intensive situations. On stud farms, increased virulence may be a factor and intensive management may substantially increase the size of the challenge, especially to the cost of weaker foals.

The virus itself can survive for nine months in the environment (which includes infected buildings) leading the way to year-on-year infection. It is also spread by healthy carriers. Mares provide some protection for their foals but this does not prevent infection where there is a heavy challenge. The virus damages the surface cells of the bowel, often leading on to problems of food absorption later.

Clinical Signs

Most affected foals are less than two months old. First signs are depression and failure to nurse, with diarrhoea appearing within 12–24 hours, watery and profuse. Fever may be the result of secondary infection. Symptoms last up to four to seven days, but diarrhoea may persist beyond this in some foals. Weight loss can be severe, but affected foals usually continue to suck. Recovered foals may shed virus for eight months.

Diagnosis

Techniques for diagnosis, based on finding virus particles in the faeces, use immunoassay, enzyme immunology, electron microscopy, and so on. Additionally, there is an ELISA test, which is the preferred method of diagnosis today. Tests must be carried out during the first few days of the illness, although it is possible for this virus to be present without causing disease. Rectal swabs from affected foals are cultured for bacterial examination where secondary infections may exist.

Treatment

Those foals badly affected require intensive fluid therapy to prevent dehydration, acidosis and electrolyte depletion. Where practical, these fluids, balanced with commercially available electrolytes, can be given orally, or even drunk from a bucket. Activated charcoal and probiotics may also be of benefit. In more severe cases, treatment may have to be given intravenously.

There is no vaccine available for use in foals, although a calf vaccine has been used to immunise mares with success. Plasma from these mares may be collected and given to infected foals by mouth – although local reactions to the vaccine may be severe in some mares.

Other Causes of Diahorrea

Nutritional diarrhoeas are caused by ingestion of excessive amounts of fibrous material or milk (weak foals with very milky dams, or foals on foster mothers, may scour from too much milk), ingestion of sand or dirt and carbohydrate intolerance. Where there is excessive milk intake, as with a fostered foal, the excessive amount may arrive undigested in the large bowel and cause diarrhoea. Lactose intolerance occurs as a clinical entity and leads to malabsorption, possibly after viral diarrhoea of foals.

Lactose in mare's milk is digested by foals through the use of lactase (an enzyme) though this gradually disappears as animals grow older. An absence of this enzyme from the foal's intestine will lead to scouring and lactose fed to adult horses is unlikely to be digested and will ferment.

Diarrhoea from *S. westeri* is thought unlikely from a milk source because of the likely level of infection; though some opinion suggests that contamination of the dam's udder and local environment with infective larvae may provoke foaling-heat diarrhoea.

Chronic diarrhoea often evolves from the acute condition, especially in Thoroughbred foals, and this might be precipitated by stress. It could also be due to heavy feeding with associated bowel damage. Worms might also be a factor, and there is often an increase of protozoa in the faeces.

If the animal is thriving, despite the diarrhoea, it is best to observe and ensure adequate fluid intake. If it is not, the use of a compatible plasma may provide a stimulus, and B vitamins may help by injection.

Strongylus vulgaris may be a cause of diarrhoea and colic in foals between one and three months of age, on worm-sick paddocks. The foal may have a temperature and signs occur suddenly. There may also be abdomominal distension and tenesmus. Very often, foals scouring from worms do so before the infection is patent.

Gastric and Duodenal Ulcers

There is an increasing incidence of gastric and duodenal ulcers and the reasons have to be assimilated. This is especially true if the incidence is management provoked, or is capable of being prevented by improved management techniques.

Occurring in foals of all ages, the clinical signs of duodenal ulcers are basically the same as they are for gastric ulcers. Indeed, there may be duodenal and gastric ulcers at the same time. Gastric ulcers that develop secondary to duodenal ulcers are associated with gastro-oesophageal reflux and oesophagitis.

Causes

Foals are able to secrete gastric acid as early as two days old. It has been suggested that the problem of ulcers may arise from immature regulation of acid secretion and incompletely developed mucosal protective processes, particularly in the gastric glandular and duodenal mucosa.

Stress is thought to be a contributing factor.

The cause could be infectious though no specific pathogen has been recognised to date. The part played by rotavirus has been considered where it occurs on a herd basis. A reported case in the United Kingdom has been associated with *Campylobacter jejuni*. In the United States, an association with over-feeding mares in pregnancy has been suggested.

NSAIDs are a known cause of ulceration. Duodenal ulcers are more likely to lead to perforation with peritonitis and adhesions, stricture of the duodenum, perhaps causing complete or partial obstruction, and ascending cholangitis and hepatitis. Lesions appear in the proximal duodenum and vary from diffuse inflammation to focal bleeding ulcers.

Clinical Signs

The first noticed sign may be bruxism (grinding of the teeth). There may be colic-type pain after sucking, and ptyalism (drooling) is a frequent sign. There may be a reluctance to suck, or complete anorexia. The foal may lie in dorsal recumbency. Signs of salivation or oesophageal reflux may indicate gastric outlet obstruction, and may be associated with ulceration of the pylorus or duodenum or both. Most affected foals have lesions along the greater curvature of the stomach. Many of these show no symptoms, though this will depend on the extent of the lesion and its situation. There may be diarrhoea, poor growth, poor coat and a pot belly.

In many foals, ulcers of the stomach resolve of their own accord and do not require treatment. In others, large, invasive ulcers may lead to haemorrhage, and diarrhoea is likely. These cases often occur in foals under two months of age.

In foals older than three months, the tendency is for ulcers to be more extensive and more widespread and for clinical signs to be more apparent.

Gastric ulcers in foals may result in substantial blood loss, causing anaemia and hypoproteinaemia, though this mostly occurs only in younger foals. Perforation may sometimes occur without prior warning and foals may be found acutely distressed or even dead. Most foals with perforations have peritonitis and many peforations occur along the lesser curvature of the stomach. Ulcers are unusual in foals less than two weeks old.

Ulcers are associated with recurrent colic, weight loss, anorexia and diarrhoea. There may be delayed gastric emptying (gauged by clearance of barium).

Diagnosis

There can be difficulties in diagnosis. Endoscopy is the most positive approach and the best means of diagnosis. It may be warranted where symptoms suggest the existence of ulcers and perhaps where faecal examination reveals the presence of occult blood. Other methods include radiography and laboratory examination of peritoneal fluid.

Before endoscopy takes place, foals up to three weeks old would have sucked but have no solid feed for ten hours. Older foals and adult horses should not have fed for ten hours so as to ensure an empty stomach. The stomach is insufflated with air to make the surfaces visible. A 200cm endoscope is required to enter the duodenum of foals. The presence of bile-tinged reflux material in the animal's stomach is not looked on as being abnormal.

While the diet is milk only, this fact will be reflected in the intestinal contents. Variations from normal might indicate excessive milk intake, foal-heat scour, and the like.

Gastric juice may be taken and examined from animals starved for 24 hours. A reading of pH 1.5–2.0 is normal for the empty stomach but would rise to pH 4.0–6.0 in the presence of food. The presence of blood may indicate ulcers.

Treatment

Controlling intake may resolve the problem over a period of weeks if there has been no permanent damage or stricture resulting from the ulcers.

Antacids should not be given liberally because the acid of the stomach helps protect the tract from pathogenic organisms.

New drugs are being developed to control gastric acid production of horses and are likely to be much better than those already being used.

Colonic and Anal Atresia

As hereditary or congenital conditions, both colonic and anal atresia occur in foals. These are expressed as non-development of parts of the tract causing partial or complete blockage. In severe cases, surgery may be required to establish patency. Some cases of atresia ani respond well to minor local surgery; others cannot be successfully treated.

Umbilical Hernia

A common birth defect of foals, umbilical hernia may be extensive, depending on the size of the abdominal fault. Most cases lend themselves to surgical repair, although minor hernias frequently disappear as the foal develops, without any need for interference.

Cleft Palate

Foals may be born with cleft soft palate and return milk down the nose; the problem is corrected surgically in some cases.

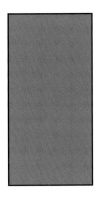

Glossary

abscess	localised collection of pus
absorption	way in which products of digestion enter the body
absorption test	to check the efficiency of the gut
acetic acid	saturated fatty acid
acid-base balance	state of equilibrium between acidity and alkalinity of the blood and body fluids
acidosis	excessive acid in blood and body fluids
activated charcoal	organic residue used to protect inflamed bowel and absorb toxins
acute disease	has sudden onset and short course
adenosine triphosphate (ATP)	energy store present in all cells
adhesion	union of two normally separate surfaces
adrenal gland	hormone-producing gland located near the kidney
aerobic	organism (or biological process) needing oxygen to function fully
aflatoxin	toxic product of fungus *Aspergillus flavus*
albumin	a protein concerned with osmotic pressure of blood
aldosterone	hormone of the adrenal gland
alkali reserve	the capacity of substances like bicarbonate to neutralise blood acid
alkaline phosphatase (AP)	enzyme of cell membranes detected in blood serum in some diseases
alkaloid	plant-derived (sometimes synthetic) therapeutic substance of the nature of morphine, atropine, quinine

alkalosis	excessive base or alkali in blood and body fluids
allergy	tissue reaction based on prior exposure to an antigen
aloin	purgative for horses (no longer in common use)
aluminium hydroxide	antacid used against ulcers
amino acid	principal breakdown constituent of protein
amylase	enzyme involved in breakdown of starch
anaemia	subnormal number of red cells or haemoglobin in blood
anaerobe	organism that lives in absence of oxygen
anaphylaxis	exaggerated allergic reaction, may be local or generalised
aneurysm	dilatation of blood vessel wall
anorexia	loss of appetite
antacid	agent to counter acidity
antibody	protein produced by lymphocyte cells against antigen, like virus, bacteria
antitoxin	antibody produced against a toxin
arginase (ARG)	liver enzyme released in disease of that organ
articular cartilage	covers surface of synovial joint
arytenoid	cartilage of the larynx
ascites	accumulation of serous fluid in peritoneal cavity
aspartate aminotransferase (AST)	enzyme found in heart, muscle and liver
ataxia	lack of muscular coordination
atonic	lacking tone
atresia ani	failure of normal anal opening to form
Bacillus piliformis	cause of Tyzzer's disease
bacteraemia	presence of bacteria in blood
bacteriocin	antibacterial substance produced by normal bowel flora
bacterium	single-celled microorganism
bile	yellowish fluid produced by liver
bile duct	channel transporting bile from liver to duodenum
bilirubin	bile pigment resulting from breakdown of haemoglobin

biopsy	tissue removed from body for examination
blowfly	insect that lays larvae on damaged areas of skin
bolus	ball of food about to be swallowed
bot	maggot of fly, found in horse's stomach
botulism	mostly fatal disease caused by bacterial poison
bracken	poisonous fern
bran disease	bone changes caused by excessive dietary phosphorus when feeding only bran
bromsulphalein (BSP)	compound used in liver function test
buckwheat	a cause of photosensitization
buffer	substance in solution that alters alkalinity or acidity
butyric acid	saturated fatty acid
caecum	first part of large intestine
calculus	abnormal concretion, like gallstone or kidney stone
Campylobacter	bacterium, capable of causing bowel infection
canine tooth	long tooth situated between molars and incisors in each jaw
cantharidin	used as blister, extracted from the blister beetle
cap	remains of milk tooth on top of erupting permanent tooth
carbohydrate	food energy source, consisting of carbon, hydrogen and oxygen
cardiac muscle	type of muscle found in heart
carotenoid pigment	yellow pigment found in carrots and green leaves
cascara sagrada	a cathartic
castor oil	a purgative
catabolism	breakdown of complex substances with production of energy
cathartic	agent causing bowel evacuation
cellulose	carbohydrate found in plant cells
cestoda	class to which tapeworms belong
chloride	anion of extracellular fluid, gastric juice
chlorine	chemical used as disinfectant

chlorophyll	green pigment involved in metabolism of plants
cholangitis	inflammation of bile duct
cholecystokinin (CCK)	hormone of small intestine
cholelithiasis	presence of gallstones in gall bladder or bile duct
cholesterol	alcohol found in all body cells
chronic	persistent or slow-developing disease
chyle	milky fluid absorbed from intestine during digestion
chyme	food mixture entering small intestine from stomach
cirrhosis	disease marked by hardening of liver
Clostridium botulinum	bacterial cause of botulism
Clostridium perfringens	bacterium sometimes associated with bowel disease
colic	pain of abdominal origin
colicin	product of *E. coli* capable of destroying other bacteria
colon	large intestine from caecum to rectum
colostrum	first milk, sometimes released before foaling
coma	deep unconscious state
concentrate	concentrated food, designed to reduce bulk and increase quality
connective tissue	fibrous tissue that connects organs, forms bones, etc.
constipation	delayed digestion time marked by hard faeces
contrast medium	material used to visualise internal organs in radiography
convulsion	involuntary contraction of muscle seen in some nervous diseases
cortex	outer layer of some organs; for example kidney, adrenal gland
cortisol	hormone of adrenal cortex
cortisone	steroid isolated from adrenal cortex
culture medium	substance used for growth of living cells, like bacteria
cutaneous habronemiasis	skin disease caused by *Habronema* species
Cyathostomum	worm member of small strongyles

cyst	fluid containing sac or capsule
deglutition	act of swallowing
dehydration	abnormal loss of body fluid
dermatitis	inflammation of skin
desquamate	shedding of cells, from skin, bowel surface, etc.
detoxify	remove toxic properties
diabetes mellitus	disease marked by low blood glucose, frequent urination, excessive thirst
diaphragm	divides abdomen from chest cavity
diaphragmatic flutter	violent repetitive hiccoughs seen sometimes in extreme exhaustion
diarrhoea	excessively watery faeces
Dicrocoelium	a type of fluke
digesta	food material during process of digestion
digestion	process of converting food into form that can be used by body
dihydroxyanthraquinone	product of dye industry used as purgative
dilatation	stretched beyond normal
dung beetle	beetle invader of faecal material on ground
duodenum	first part of small intestine
dysphagia	difficulty in swallowing
electrolyte	chemical substances which dissociate into positive and negative ions when dissolved in water; for example (Na+) (Cl-), components of sodium chloride (NaCl)
electron microscope	uses short wavelength electron beam for illumination; 100 times stronger than light microscope
ELISA	enzyme-linked immunosorbent assay for detecting antibodies or antigens
embolus	blood clot blocking artery
emphysema	abnormal presence of air in tissues
emulsion	mixture of two immiscible liquids
encysted	enclosed in a sac
endocrine	secreting internally
endogenous	produced within
endoscope	instrument for inspection of internal organs
endotoxaemia	presence of endotoxins in blood

endotoxin	toxin present in bacterial cell wall
energy	product of chemical reactions allowing for movement, heat production, etc.
enteritis	inflammation of intestine
enterocolitis	inflammation of small intestine and colon
enterokinase	intestinal hormone
enterotoxic	toxin damaging to intestinal cells
enzyme	protein catalyst increasing rate of chemical reaction
Epicauta vittata	the blister beetle
epiglottis	cartilage at entrance to larynx
epinephrine	also adrenalin, hormone of the adrenal medulla
epiphysis	end of long bone
epistaxis	bleeding from nose
erythema	redness of skin
Escherichia (E.) *coli*	bacterium inhabiting bowel
exercise tolerance	ability to withstand work
exhaustion	depletion of energy
exocrine	secretes externally through a duct
exogenous	originating outside
extracellular fluid	body fluid existing outside cells
exudate	discharge as might come from a wound or inflamed tissue
Fagopyrum saggittatum	buckwheat, cause of photosensitization
fascia	fibrous tissue helping to bind muscles, etc.
Fasciola hepatica	liver fluke
fat	adipose tissue of body
fat-soluble vitamin	absorbed from intestine dissolved in fat
fatty acid	compound of carbon, hydrogen and oxygen that combines with glycerol to form fat
fatty infiltration	invasion of tissue with fat
fermentation	part of digestive process in large bowel for breaking down complex carbohydrates to simple sugars
fibre	part of diet containing structural carbohydrates, as in hay, chaff, essential to normal working of the large bowel
fibrinogen	protein found in plasma, essential to clotting

flexural deformity	fixed joints in newborn foals, usually with contracted tendons
flora	normal resident organisms of bowel
fluke	leaf-shaped parasite of liver
flunixin meglumine	non-steroidal anti-inflammatory agent
forage	processed winter feed like hay, silage
frenum linguae	anatomical attachment of tongue to floor of mouth
fundus	bottom, or base, of an organ
fungus	group of organisms including moulds, yeasts, mushrooms
gallstone	stone that forms in gall bladder or bile duct
Gasterophilus intestinalis	horse bot fly
gastric juice	secretion of glands in stomach
gastrin	hormone produced in the stomach
glottis	vocal apparatus of larynx
glucagon	hormone involved in glucose metabolism
glucocorticoid	substance involved in glucose metabolism; also used widely as an anti-inflammatory agent
glucose	simple sugar, major source of energy
glutathione peroxidase	enzyme used to indicate selenium levels of animals
glycogen	substance through which carbohydrate is stored in animal
glycosuria	presence of glucose in urine
goitre	enlargement of thyroid gland
gram negative	reaction to stain used to identify bacteria
growth plate	part of epiphysis involved in growth of long bones
haemaglobinuria	presence of haemaglobin in urine
haematoma	localised collection of blood; a blood blister
haemolysis	rupture of red blood cells
haemolytic anaemia	anaemia caused by excessive destruction of red blood cells
haemotology	study of blood
hard palate	bony roof of mouth
Helicobacter	organism associated with human stomach ulcers

Heliotropium europaeum	heliotrope, cause of photosensitization
heparin	substance present in many living tissues, also used as anticoagulant
hepatitis	inflammation of liver
hernia	abnormal protrusion of organ (or part of) through surrounding tissues
hydration	provision of water, as in body water balance
hyoid apparatus	suspensory mechanism for tongue and larynx
hyperglycaemia	excess of glucose in blood
Hypericum perfoliatum	St John's wort, a cause of photosensitization
hyperlipaemia	excess of fat in blood
hypertrophy	increase in size of an organ
hypocalcaemia	inadequate calcium in blood
hypoglycaemia	inadequate glucose in blood
hypoproteinaemia	inadequate protein in blood
hypovolaemia	abnormally low volume of circulating body fluid
hypoxia	inadequate oxygen for body tissues
ileum	last part of small intestine
ileus	failure of peristalsis
immunoassay	measurement of antibody or antigen
immunodeficiency	lack of immune response
immunoglobulin	type of antibody
impaction	blockage
inappetance	partial lack of appetite
incisor	cutting tooth, situated at front of mouth
infarct	local area of dead tissue resulting from interference with blood supply
inflammation	tissue response to injury or disease
ingesta	food material taken by mouth into body
inguinal	relating to the groin
injected membranes	inflamed or flushed membranes
insulin	pancreatic hormone involved in glucose metabolism
intercellular	between cells
intermediate host	essential carrier of parasite or infection
intracellular	within cells

intraluminal	within lumen, as in centre of bowel
jaundice	denoted by yellow mucous membranes, sign of liver disease
jejunum	section of small intestine between duodenum and ileum
ketone bodies	normal breakdown products of fat metabolism
lactase	intestinal enzyme breaking down lactose
lactation	production of milk by mammary gland, or period from start to finish of milk production
lactic acid	compound resulting from carbohydrate metabolism
lactobacillus	bacterium producing lactic acid by fermentation
lactose intolerance	inability to digest lactose
laminitis	condition marked by pain and heat in feet
larva	stage in life-cycle of parasite or insect
larynx	called the 'voice-box', structure made of cartilage joining pharynx and trachea
latent	dormant, in wait
laxative	medicine encouraging bowel evacuation
lignin	indigestible carbohydrate found in straw and wool
lipase	enzyme breaking down fats
lipid	fat or wax found in living cells
local pH	acidity or alkalinity of medium, perhaps within section of bowel
lymph	yellowish fluid contained within lymphatic vessels
lymph node	small glandular structures found on course of lymph vessels, often enlarged in infection
lymphoid tissue	tissue of lymphatic system
lysozyme	antibacterial enzyme found in tears, saliva, etc.
magnesium sulphate	Epsom salts, used as cathartic
malabsorption	failure of intestine to absorb nutrients

maltose	sugar derived from starch
mandible	bone of lower jaw
maxilla	bone of upper jaw
meconium	first faeces of foal
melanin	dark pigment found in hair, skin, etc.
mesentery	sheet of peritoneum attaching intestine to abdominal wall
metabolism	process converting food into living tissue, its maintenance, energy production and breakdown
methane	gas produced from decomposition of organic matter
methionine	sulphur containing essential amino acid
microbial digestion	digestion of food by organisms
microfilaria	worm larva transmitted by intermediate host
milk teeth	first or temporary teeth
molar	last three cheek teeth on each jaw
morbidity	in diseased condition
morbidity rate	percentage of diseased to healthy animals in a population, especially relating to specific disease entity
mortality rate	death rate in disease incident
motility	with spontaneous movement
mould	fungus causing furry growth on organic matter
mucosa	mucous membrane
mucous membrane	membrane covered with epithelium that produces mucus
mucus	sticky secretion of mucosal glands
mycotoxicosis	poisoning from fungal toxin
nasopharynx	part of pharynx above soft palate
necrosis	cell death
necrotizing enteritis	inflammation of intestine with cell death
Nematoda	class of roundworm
nephrosplenic ligament	section of peritoneum between spleen and left kidney
norepinephrine	(also called noradrenaline) hormone that affects heart rate, blood pressure, etc.
NSAID	non-steroidal anti-inflammatory drug

obligate anaerobe	organism that can only grow in absence of oxygen
obstruction	blockage
occult	obscure or hidden
oedema	abnormal presence of fluid in cavities or intercellular tissues
oesophagitis	inflammation of oesophagus
oesophagus	tubular organ extending between pharynx and stomach
organophosphate	potentially poisonous compound used as insecticide and anthelmintic
oribatid mite	intermediate host of tapeworm
oropharynx	part of pharynx between soft palate, tongue and epiglottis
osmosis	way in which matter passes across membrane in solution
osteodystrophia fibrosa	*see* bran disease
osteomalacia	softening of bone due to failed mineralisation
oxalate	poisonous plant substance adversely affecting calcium absorption
Oxalis acetosella	wood sorrel, contains high oxalate content
Oxyuris equi	roundworm causing irritation of anus
palatine bone	bone of hard palate
palpate	to handle
pancreatic fluid	digestive liquid produced by the pancreas
pancreatitis	inflammation of pancreas
pancreozymin-cholecystokinin	hormone of duodenal mucosa helping pancreatic secretion
paracentesis	surgical collection of fluid from cavity
Parascaris equorum	horse roundworm
parathormone	hormone of parathyroid gland
parotid gland	salivary gland situated near ear
pathogen	disease-producing organism or agent
pathology	study of disease effects on organs and tissues
pelvis	bony girdle formed by ilium, ischium, pubic bones and sacrum
Penicillium	type of fungus
pepsin	gastric enzyme involved in protein digestion

pepsinogen	precursor of pepsin
perineum	hairless region around anus and genital organs
periosteum	outer layer of bone
peristalsis	movement of bowel that propels food along
peritonitis	inflammation of peritoneum
petechiae	pinpoint haemorrhages
pH	measure of alkalinity or acidity of a solution
pharynx	throat
phenothiazine	outdated wormer, capable of causing photosensitization
phenylbutazone	a non-steroidal anti-inflammatory drug
phospholipid	lipid that contains phosphorus
photodynamic substance	substance activated by light to cause tissue damage
photosensitization	reaction to sunlight of skin primed by photodynamic substance
phytase	enzyme involved in breakdown of phytate
phytate	dietary source of phosphorus
placental transfer	refers to transfer of antibodies from dam to foal *in utero*
plasma cell	type of cell associated with antibody production
plasma viscosity	characteristic of blood measurement which may indicate disease, or altered protein level
prehension	to grasp, used in relation to eating
premaxilla	bone at front of hard palate
premolar tooth	first three molar teeth on each jaw
probiotic	substance favouring normal gut flora
proglottid	tapeworm segment
prolapse	describes displacement of organ, for example of rectum or uterus externally
propionate	a salt of propionic acid
propionic acid	volatile fatty acid that breaks down to produce glucose
protein	compound of carbon, hydrogen, oxygen and nitrogen made from chains of amino acids
proteolytic	breaks down protein

prothrombin	a protein involved in blood clotting
protozoa	division of single-celled organism that can cause disease; includes coccidia
pruritis	itchiness
psyllium hydrophilic mucilloid	bulk mild cathartic
ptyalism	excessive salivation
pubis	front bone of the pelvis
pulse	heart beat felt through arterial wall
purgative	agent to cause bowel evacuation
putrefaction	decomposition
pylorus	stomach opening into duodenum
rabies	usually fatal virus disease affecting nervous system
rancid	rank-smelling decomposed fat
rectum	terminal segment of bowel
red blood cell	oxygen-carrying cell of blood
reflux	returned flow, referring to food content of stomach or intestine
regurgitate	return of food into mouth; may be normal as with ruminants chewing cud
renal	relating to kidney
Rhodococcus equi	bacterial cause of chronic pneumonia and enteritis in foals
rickets	improper bone development due to deficiency of phosphorus or vitamin D
rotavirus	viral cause of sometimes epidemic diarrhoea in foals
roundworm	worms of the class Nematoda mostly infecting digestive system when mature
rubratoxin	fungal toxin causing liver damage
sacculation	formed into pouches, or sacs
saline	refers to salt solution, as in 'normal saline' used in intravenous fluid replacement therapy
saliva	secretion of salivary glands
salivary gland	any of a number of glands in region of mouth producing saliva
Salmonella	bacterial cause of diarrhoea in horses of all ages

scan	refers to image production – using diagnostic ultrasound, for example
secrete	release of liquid product
secretin	hormone produced in duodenum
Senecio jacobea	ragwort, poisonous plant causing liver damage
senna	a cathartic
septicaemia	disease condition marked by presence of bacteria in blood
serology	laboratory examination of antibody-antigen reactions
serotonin	hormone inhibiting gastric secretion as well as other actions
serous membrane	membrane secreting a watery fluid
serum	fluid of blood after clotting
skeletal muscle	muscle of the skeleton
sloughed skin	dead skin that peels off
soft palate	fleshy backward extension from hard palate
spleen	organ located to left of stomach that acts as reserve of red blood cells, especially in athletic animal
starch	chief storage form of carbohydrates in plants
steatorrhoea	excess fat in faeces
sternum	the breastbone
steroid hormone	includes male and female sex hormones, also cortisone, etc.
stomach	enlargement of digestive tract between oesophagus and duodenum
strangles	bacterial disease marked by discharging glands
strangulation	refers to restriction of blood supply to bowel segment
Streptococcus equi	bacterial cause of strangles
stricture	refers to abnormal narrowing of bowel segment
Strongyloides westeri	roundworm, larvae of which may be passed to foal in milk
Strongylus vulgaris	a large strongyle worm
structural carbohydrate	complex carbohydrates subject to bacterial digestion in large bowel

subacute	between acute and chronic
sublingual gland	salivary gland situated beneath tongue
submaxillary gland	salivary gland beneath maxilla
Succus entericus	secretion of intestinal glands
sucrose	sugar produced from beet, sugar cane
sulphonamide	antibacterial drug
summer sores	sweet itch, etc.
symbiosis	mutually beneficial co-existence, as where gut bacteria benefit host through food digestion
systemic infection	affects general body systems
tenesmus	straining
tetanus	often fatal bacterial disease of nervous system caused by *Clostridium tetani*
tetany	clinical syndrome marked by rigidity of limbs
thorax	the chest cavity
thyroid gland	hormone-producing gland of upper neck
thyroxine	a hormone of the thyroid
tongue	muscular organ on floor of mouth
torsion	act of twisting
toxaemia	presence of toxins in blood
toxigenic	produces toxin
toxin	poison produced by plants, bacteria, etc.
trace element	essential dietary elements required only in small amounts
Trematoda	class of worm to which liver fluke belongs
Trichostrongylus axei	roundworm affecting cattle, sheep and horses
triglyceride	usual form of fat storage in animals
trypsin	enzyme involved in protein digestion
trypsinogen	precursor of trypsin, secreted by pancreas
tumour	usually refers to cancerous growth
tying-up	disease syndrome marked by stiffening during or after exercise
Tyzzer's disease	fatal bacterial liver disease caused by *Bacillus piliformis*
ulcer	tissue defect resulting from cell death

ultrasound	equipment used for diagnosis and therapy, based on transmission of sound waves
umbilicus	remnant of foetal attachment to dam *in utero*
unsaturated fatty acid	liquid at room temperature and found in linseed oil, olive oil
urea	chief nitrogenous end-product of protein metabolism
urease	enzyme involved in breakdown of urea
vector	refers to insect disease carrier
villus	hair-like process on surface cell
virulence	ability of infectious agent to cause disease
viscera	refers to abdominal organs
vitamin	organic substance essential to life
vocal fold	part of larynx associated with voice
volatile fatty acid	breakdown product of cellulose digestion in large bowel
vomit	emission of food material from stomach – via nostril, in case of horse
white blood cell	disease-fighting cell of blood
wolf tooth	rudimentary tooth situated in front of first premolar in upper jaw of horses
xylose	sugar used in absorption test
yeast	a type of fungus

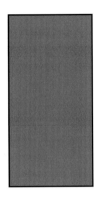

Index